Immunology: Function, Pathology, Diagnostics, and Modulation

Guest Editor

MELISSA A. KENNEDY, DVM, PhD

VETERINARY CLINICS OF NORTH AMERICA: SMALL ANIMAL PRACTICE

www.vetsmall.theclinics.com

May 2010 • Volume 40 • Number 3

SAUNDERS an imprint of ELSEVIER, Inc.

W.B. SAUNDERS COMPANY
A Division of Elsevier Inc.

1600 John F. Kennedy Blvd. ● Suite 1800 ● Philadelphia, PA 19103-2899

http://www.vetsmall.theclinics.com

VETERINARY CLINICS OF NORTH AMERICA: SMALL ANIMAL PRACTICE Volume 40, Number 3
May 2010 ISSN 0195-5616, ISBN-13: 978-1-4377-1888-1

Editor: John Vassallo; j.vassallo@elsevier.com

Veterinary Clinics of North America: Small Animal Practice (ISSN 0195-5616) is published bimonthly (For Post Office use only: volume 40 issue 3 of 6) by Elsevier Inc., 360 Park Avenue South, New York, NY 10010-1710. Months of issue are January, March, May, July, September, and November. Business and Editorial Offices: 1600 John F. Kennedy Blvd., Ste. 1800, Philadelphia, PA 19103-2899. Customer Service Office: 3251 Riverport Lane, Maryland Heights, MO 63043. Periodicals postage paid at New York, NY and additional mailing offices. Subscription prices are $245.00 per year (domestic individuals), $388.00 per year (domestic institutions), $122.00 per year (domestic students/residents), $324.00 per year (Canadian individuals), $477.00 per year (Canadian institutions), $360.00 per year (international individuals), $477.00 per year (international institutions), and $177.00 per year (international and Canadian students/residents). To receive student/resident rate, orders must be accompanied by name of affiliated institution, date of term, and the *signature* of program/residency coordinator on institution letterhead. Orders will be billed at individual rate until proof of status is received. Foreign air speed delivery is included in all *Clinics* subscription prices. All prices are subject to change without notice. **POSTMASTER:** Send address changes to *Veterinary Clinics of North America: Small Animal Practice*, Elsevier Health Sciences Division, Subscription Customer Service, 3251 Riverport Lane, Maryland Heights, MO 63043. Customer Service (orders, claims, on-line, change of address): Elsevier Periodicals Customer Service, Elsevier Health Sciences Division Subscription Customer Service 3251 Riverport Lane Maryland Heights, MO 63043. Tel: 1-800-654-2452 (U.S. and Canada); 314-447-8871 (outside U.S. and Canada). Fax: 314-447-8029. E-mail: journalscustomerservice-usa@elsevier.com (for print support); journalsonlinesupport-usa@elsevier.com (for online support).

Reprints. For copies of 100 or more of articles in this publication, please contact the Commercial Reprints Department, Elsevier Inc., 360 Park Avenue South, New York, NY 10010-1710. Tel.: 212-633-3812; Fax: 212-462-1935; E-mail: reprints@elsevier.com.

Veterinary Clinics of North America: Small Animal Practice is also published in Japanese by Inter Zoo Publishing Co., Ltd., Aoyama Crystal-Bldg 5F, 3-5-12 Kitaaoyama, Minato-ku, Tokyo 107-0061, Japan.

Veterinary Clinics of North America: Small Animal Practice is covered in *Current Contents/Agriculture, Biology and Environmental Sciences, Science Citation Index, ASCA, MEDLINE/PubMed (Index Medicus), Excerpta Medica,* and *BIOSIS.*

Printed and bound by CPI Group (UK) Ltd, Croydon, CR0 4YY

Transferred to Digital Print 2011

Contributors

GUEST EDITOR

MELISSA A. KENNEDY, DVM, PhD
Diplomate, American College of Veterinary Internal Medicine; Associate Professor,
Department of Comparative Medicine, College of Veterinary Medicine, University
of Tennessee, Knoxville, Tennessee

AUTHORS

PHILIP J. BERGMAN, DVM, MS, PhD
Diplomate, American College of Veterinary Internal Medicine (Oncology); Chief Medical
Officer, BrightHeart Veterinary Centers, Armonk; Adjunct Associate Member,
Memorial Sloan-Kettering Cancer Center, New York, New York

CRAIG A. DATZ, DVM, MS
Diplomate, American Board of Veterinary Practitioners; Assistant Professor, Department
of Veterinary Medicine and Surgery, College of Veterinary Medicine, University of Missouri,
Columbia, Missouri

MARY C. DEBEY, DVM, PhD
Diplomate, American College of Veterinary Microbiologists; Consultation Clinician,
Hill's Veterinary Consultation Service, Hill's Pet Nutrition, Inc, Topeka, Kansas

LAUREL J. GERSHWIN, DVM, PhD
Diplomate, American College of Veterinary Microbiology; Professor of Immunology,
Service Chief for Clinical Immunology, Department of Pathology, Microbiology, and
Immunology, Veterinary Medical Teaching Hospital, School of Veterinary Medicine,
University of California, Davis, California

HARM HOGENESCH, DVM, PhD
Diplomate, American College of Veterinary Pathologists; Department of Comparative
Pathobiology, School of Veterinary Medicine, Purdue University, West Lafayette, Indiana

STEPHEN A. KANIA, PhD
Associate Professor, Department of Comparative Medicine, College of Veterinary
Medicine, University of Tennessee, Knoxville, Tennessee

MELISSA A. KENNEDY, DVM, PhD
Diplomate, American College of Veterinary Internal Medicine; Associate Professor,
Department of Comparative Medicine, College of Veterinary Medicine,
University of Tennessee, Knoxville, Tennessee

SCOTT MCVEY, DVM, PhD
Diplomate, American College of Veterinary Microbiologists; School of Veterinary Medicine
and Biomedical Sciences, College of Agriculture and Natural Resources, Nebraska
Veterinary Diagnostic Center, University of Nebraska-Lincoln, Lincoln, Nebraska

GEORGE E. MOORE, DVM, MS, PhD
Department of Comparative Pathobiology, School of Veterinary Medicine,
Purdue University, West Lafayette, Indiana

BARRAK M. PRESSLER, DVM, PhD
Diplomate, American College of Veterinary Internal Medicine (Small Animal Internal
Medicine); Assistant Professor of Small Animal Internal Medicine, Department
of Veterinary Clinical Sciences, School of Veterinary Medicine, Purdue University,
West Lafayette, Indiana

JISHU SHI, DVM, PhD
Department of Anatomy and Physiology, College of Veterinary Medicine,
Kansas State University, Manhattan, Kansas

JANE E. SYKES, BVSc(Hons), PhD
Diplomate, American College of Veterinary Internal Medicine; Associate Professor
of Small Animal Internal Medicine, Department of Medicine and Epidemiology,
University of California, Davis, California

EILEEN L. THACKER, DVM, PhD
National Program Leader, Animal Health, United States Department of Agriculture -
Agricultural Research Service, Beltsville, Maryland

LYNEL J. TOCCI, DVM, MT(ASCP)SBB
Department Head, Department of Emergency and Critical Care, Veterinary Emergency
and Specialty Center of New England, Waltham, Massachusetts

Contents

The role of the immune system is simple yet challenging: to eliminate pathogenic agents. The immune system contains nonspecific and specific components; that is, some constituents act without precise recognition of the target, others have exquisite specificity. Regulation of the immune response and maintenance of tolerance to self are critical to the health of the animal. To properly evaluate or control immune function, knowledge of the basic components of the normal immune system is essential. This review covers the current knowledge of individual components of the immune system and how they interact to protect the host from infectious disease agents.

The use of vaccines in veterinary medicine has progressed from an experimental adventure to a routine and relatively safe practice. The common and aggressive use of efficacious vaccines has been responsible for the control and eradication of several diseases. Despite progress in research technologies, diagnostic capabilities, and manufacturing methods, there remain many infectious diseases for which no effective vaccines exist. Global availability, field compliance, effectiveness, and safety are also significant concerns. This review addresses the history, current practices, and potential future improvements of vaccine use in veterinary medicine.

Adverse vaccinal events, or perceived vaccine-associated adverse events, are relatively uncommon in companion animal practice. These events, however, often evoke great concern to owners and veterinarians. Because of the low incidence of these events and the large number of potential antigenic causes, exact mechanisms are often difficult to elucidate. This article reviews current evidence related to the immunologic basis of adverse events seen after canine and feline vaccination.

Immunodeficiencies caused by infectious agents may result from disruption of normal host barriers or dysregulation of cellular immunity, the latter serving to promote survival of the infectious agent through immune evasion. Such infections may be followed by opportunistic infections with a variety of other microorganisms. Classic infectious causes of immunodeficiency in companion animals are the immunodeficiency retroviruses, including feline immunodeficiency virus and feline leukemia virus. Other important causes include canine distemper virus; canine parvovirus 2; feline infectious perito-nitis virus; rickettsial organisms that infect leukocytes; *Leishmania*; and fun-gal pathogens, such as *Cryptococcus*. Considerable research effort has been invested in understanding the mechanisms of pathogen-induced immunosuppression, with the hope that effective therapies may be devel-oped that reverse the immunodeficiencies developed and in turn assist the host to clear persistent or life-threatening infectious diseases.

Primary immunodeficiencies are congenital defects that affect formation or function of the immune system. Congenital immunodeficiency should be considered as a differential diagnosis for repeated infections in a young animal. Defects in the immune system may lead to complete or partial loss of immunity. Some animals with mild immunodeficiency can be man-aged with long-term antibiotic therapy.

There are many autoimmune diseases recognized in humans; many of these have counterparts in companion animals. The diseases discussed in this ar-ticle do not constitute the entire spectrum of autoimmune disease in these species. They are the common and better-described diseases of dogs and cats that have a well-documented autoimmune etiology. There are myriad autoimmune diseases that affect humans; similar diseases yet unrecognized in companion animals likely will be characterized in the future. The role of genetics in predisposition to autoimmunity is a common characteristic of these diseases in humans and animals. Likewise, the suggested role of environmental or infectious agents is another commonality between humans and their pets.

Dogs and cats may be affected with primary (inherited) or secondary (ac-quired) immunodeficiency. For the latter, several infectious diseases have been found to be immunosuppressive, whereas noninfectious causes are less common and not as well characterized. This review summarizes cur-rent knowledge of immunosuppression that is not associated with infec-tion. Because of limited studies performed in dogs and cats, some of the references are taken from human and laboratory animal research. Vet-erinary clinicians can gain a greater understanding of the immune system and how it is affected by various agents and disease processes.

> Several tests are available for the diagnosis of immunologic disorders with varying availability. The tests are categorized into two groups, those that examine function and those that measure physical parameters such as cell numbers or immunoglobulin concentrations. This article highlights several of these tests and describes their use in small animals.

> Immunomodulators, immunostimulants, and immunotherapies are important tools used by veterinary practitioners and researchers to control and direct the immune system of small animals. This article is an overview and summary of some of the most common immunomodulatory agents used in companion animals emphasizing steroidal and nonsteroidal agents, T-cell inhibitors, cytotoxic drugs, immunostimulators and biologic response modifying agents, and neoplasia chemotherapeutic agents.

> Red blood cell transfusions in veterinary medicine have become increasingly more common and are an integral part of lifesaving and advanced treatment of the critically ill. Common situations involving transfusions are life-threatening anemia from acute hemorrhage or surgical blood loss, hemolysis from drugs or toxins, immune-mediated diseases, severe nonregenerative conditions, and neonatal isoerythrolysis. Although transfusions can be lifesaving, they are also associated with adverse events that can be life threatening. This article reviews the principles for pretransfusion blood typing and compatibility testing and the types of transfusion reactions that exist despite test performance.

> Cell surface proteins which mediate tolerance or rejection of transplanted organs have been well characterized in people. However, despite the relative conservation of the acquired immune response in mammals, for unknown reasons dogs and cats either tolerate transplanted organs more readily or reject them more vigorously. The rejection-associated histologic changes found in human and animal grafts imply that the immune response to graft proteins is not identical amongst species. As a result few tissues or organs are routinely transplanted in client-owned dogs and cats, and larger studies are still needed to characterize chronic changes that may develop. With the continual development of new immunosuppressive drugs and refinement of existing protocols, transplantation options will hopefully increase via the use of xenograft tissues, particularly in dogs.

The veterinary oncology profession is uniquely able to contribute to the many advances that are imminent in immunotherapy. However, what works in a mouse will often not reflect the outcome in human patients with cancer. Therefore, comparative immunotherapy studies using veterinary patients may be better able to bridge murine and human studies. Many cancers in dogs and cats seem to be stronger models for their counterpart human tumors than presently available murine model systems. This author looks forward to the time when immunotherapy plays a significant role in the treatment and/or prevention of cancer in human and veterinary patients.

THE CLINICS ARE NOW AVAILABLE ONLINE!

Access your subscription at:
www.theclinics.com

Preface

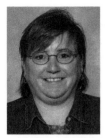

Melissa A. Kennedy, DVM, PhD
Guest Editor

The immune system is simple in its purpose—to eliminate invading pathogens—but complex in its mechanisms. It is composed of many soluble and cellular components that interact with one another to provide a formidable defense against infectious agents. The elements of the immune system vary from the physical barriers, such as the epidermis, to the most complex and specific components, the lymphocytes. Advances in the understanding of the immune response have been made, but much remains to be elucidated.

In veterinary as in human medicine, despite the gaps in understanding of the immune response, the ability to manipulate this response has been exploited for hundreds of years through vaccination. The technology involved with vaccine production has expanded from use of the killed or attenuated whole organism to molecularly developed products. The routine and aggressive use of efficacious vaccines has been, in large part, responsible for control and eradication of several diseases.

Uncommonly, adverse vaccinal events occur and, although relatively rare, evoke great concern to owners and veterinarians. Undesired biologic events can occur for myriad reasons, and cause and effect may be very difficult to determine in events following vaccination. For those definitively linked to vaccination, the mechanisms fall into one of the four hypersensitivity reactions. Other sequelae, including neoplasia, also have been linked to vaccines, but the exact mechanisms and inciting antigen are difficult to elucidate.

Regulation of the immune response and maintenance of tolerance to self antigens are critical to the health of the animal. There are situations in which an immune response may be generated such that self-tissues are attacked. These responses are referred to as autoimmune, and depending upon which of the self-antigens the immune response is directed toward, clinical signs of disease occur and are relevant to the functions of those target tissues/organs. There are several well-recognized pathogenic mechanisms for induction of autoimmune responses, and there are also many autoimmune diseases for which there is no known reason for development of the autoimmune response. The role of genetics in predisposition to autoimmunity is a common

Vet Clin Small Anim 40 (2010) xi–xiii
doi:10.1016/j.cvsm.2010.03.002
0195-5616/10/$ – see front matter © 2010 Elsevier Inc. All rights reserved.

characteristic of these diseases in people and animals. Likewise, the suggested role of environmental or infectious agents as instigating agents is another commonality between people and the pets that share their environment. Diagnosis and treatment of these conditions can be challenging.

Immunodeficiency is defined as the absence of, or decreased function of, one or more components of the immune system. Primary immunodeficiencies are congenital genetic defects that affect formation or function of cells or proteins of the immune system. These defects may affect any component of the immune system, including soluble elements, cell surface molecules, or cellular development and functions. There are likely many immunodeficiencies of dogs and cats that have not been identified.

Secondary immunodeficiencies are caused by an external influence on immune function. Numerous pathogens are capable of disrupting normal immune function. The types of opportunistic infections that occur in patients that are immune-compromised as a result of an underlying immunosuppressive infection depend upon the mechanisms of immunosuppression. Considerable research effort has been invested in understanding of the mechanisms of pathogen-induced immunosuppression, with the hope that effective therapies may be developed that reverse the immunodeficiencies developed and in turn assist the host in clearing persistent or life-threatening infectious diseases.

Various drugs, toxins, diseases, and procedures such as vaccination and anesthesia have been associated with immunosuppression in dogs and cats. Lifelong issues such as nutrition, stress, and exercise also have effects on the immune system. Veterinarians should be aware of the potential for immunodeficiency when dealing with both healthy and diseased patients. As the recognition and treatment of immunosuppression can be difficult, exposure to these noninfectious causes should be minimized or avoided if possible.

Immunologic abnormalities are often difficult to diagnose because of vague symptoms, their association with infectious diseases, and, in young animals, residual passively acquired immunity. Several tests are available for the diagnosis of immunologic disorders with varying availability. The tests are categorized into two groups, those that examine function and those that measure physical parameters such as cell numbers or immunoglobulin concentrations. Functional tests generally are less available because of issues of cell viability. Immunomodulators, immunostimulants, and immunotherapies are important tools used by veterinary practitioners and researchers to control and direct the immune system of small animals. This is a rapidly evolving field with new agents introduced, clinical trials performed, and products approved on a constant basis. Several pharmaceuticals are being tested for human use that may be useful in veterinary medicine. In addition, several natural or herbal compounds have been reported to impact the immune system; however, frequently the scientific data to support claims are not available. In recent years, new strategies targeting specific components of the immune system have been designed. These technologies have the potential of avoiding the general suppression of the immune response observed with many current conventional agents; however, even these newer drugs have adverse effects, as they affect important cells of the immune system.

Red blood cell (RBC) transfusions in veterinary medicine have become increasingly more common and are an integral part of lifesaving and advanced treatment of the critically ill. Although transfusions can be life-saving, they also are associated with adverse events that can be life-threatening. An understanding of the antigens involved, the pretransfusion testing, and the mechanisms of transfusion reactions can help to minimize adverse events.

Transplantation of a number of tissues and parenchymal organs has become an accepted treatment modality in people over the last 50 years. Despite the much more limited use of transplantation in veterinary medicine, the first reported organ transplants were performed in dogs in the early 20th century. These were followed by studies in experimental animals that demonstrated the comparative success of organ transplants from animals of the same versus different species, and refined many of the surgical techniques that are in place today. The introduction of new immunosuppressive drugs, particularly cyclosporine, in the 1980s, vastly improved both short- and long-term outcome of transplanted tissues, and thus reduced morbidity and mortality of transplant recipients. Transplantation options hopefully will increase, particularly in dogs and via the use of xenograft tissues.

Although the immune system is normally thought of as providing protection against infectious disease, the immune system's ability to recognize and eliminate cancer is the fundamental rationale for the immunotherapy of cancer. With the tools of molecular biology and a greater understanding of mechanisms to harness the immune system, effective tumor immunotherapy is becoming a reality. This new class of therapeutics offers a more targeted and therefore precise approach to the treatment of cancer. It is extremely likely that immunotherapy will have a place alongside the classic cancer treatment triad components of surgery, radiation therapy, and chemotherapy within the next 5 to 10 years.

This issue summarizes the high points of recent discoveries and advances in the understanding of the immune response, the factors that impact it, the assessment of its function, and the manipulation of the response to enhance the health of the animal.

Melissa A. Kennedy, DVM, PhD
Department of Comparative Medicine
University of Tennessee
A205 Veterinary Teaching Hospital
2407 River Drive
Knoxville, TN 37996-4543, USA

E-mail address:
mkenned2@utk.edu

A Brief Review of the Basics of Immunology: The Innate and Adaptive Response

Melissa A. Kennedy, DVM, PhD

KEYWORDS
- Immune system • Innate response
- Adaptive response • Tolerance

The role of the immune system is simple yet difficult: to eliminate pathogenic agents. The immune system contains nonspecific and specific components; that is, some constituents act without precise recognition of the target, others have exquisite specificity. Although distinct, these 2 arms interact at many levels, and the many elements of the immune system are intricately interrelated. These elements vary from the physical barriers, such as the epidermis, to the most complex and specific components, the lymphocytes. Regulation of the immune response and maintenance of tolerance to self are critical to the health of the animal. One avenue for regulation and maintenance, vaccination, uses the immune response to enhance protection of the animal. Manipulation of the response is being explored for a variety of immune-mediated and immunosuppressive diseases. To properly evaluate or control immune function, knowledge of the basic components of the normal immune system is essential. This review covers the current knowledge of individual components of the immune system and how they interact to protect the host from infectious disease agents.

OVERVIEW

The immune system can be envisaged as having 2 arms of defense, nonspecific and specific. The nonspecific arm is that with which the animal is born and does not possess specific antigenic recognition. The specific arm, as its name implies, possesses exquisite specificity of antigen recognition. Both arms involve several distinct components.

The nonspecific arm of the immune response has many elements that have in common their lack of strict recognition of foreign material and absence of memory. The nonspecific arm is also referred to as innate immunity, as it is present at birth

Department of Comparative Medicine, College of Veterinary Medicine, University of Tennessee, Room A205 VTH, 2407 River Drive, Knoxville, TN 37996-4543, USA
E-mail address: mkenned2@utk.edu

Vet Clin Small Anim 40 (2010) 369–379
doi:10.1016/j.cvsm.2010.01.003
0195-5616/10/$ – see front matter © 2010 Elsevier Inc. All rights reserved.

unlike specific acquired immunity, which develops after birth and is also known as adaptive immunity. The innate response is the first line of defense against infectious disease, and if effective, may completely eliminate the agent before the specific adaptive immune response is called on. The innate response also interacts with the adaptive immune response, aiding its activation and modulating the response.

The simplest components of the innate response to understand are the anatomic and physiologic barriers. These include the skin and mucous membranes, as well as physical parameters such as temperature, pH, and oxygen levels. These barriers are comprised not only of the cells at the surface but also soluble components, such as enzymes, antimicrobial peptides, and cytokines.

More complex, but still nonspecific in terms of antigen recognition, are the phagocytic and cytotoxic cells, as well as various soluble components .The latter elements include various antimicrobial molecules such as complement, as well as components that mediate the inflammatory processes, such as kinins, leukotrienes, and prostaglandins. Cellular components include neutrophils, eosinophils, basophils, mast cells, and natural killer (NK) lymphocytes. The first 4 types are of granulocyte lineage and possess cytosolic granules filled with enzymes and microbicidal substances; in addition, neutrophils and eosinophils are phagocytic. NK cells, although from the lymphocyte lineage, lack antigen-specific receptors on their surface, and are important mediators of cell-mediated immunity. Distinct from these cells are the monocytes/macrophages and dendritic cells. Monocytes are phagocytic cells circulating in the blood; macrophage is the term for these cells in tissue. Dendritic cells are distinct phagocytic cells found in tissue and lymphoid organs. All 3 of these cell types, in addition to phagocytosis and destruction of invading microbes, are critical to the specific immune response. In particular, dendritic cells are integral to an effective and appropriate immune response.

The specific immune response involves lymphocytes, the only cells that possess specificity, diversity of recognition, and memory.[1] The lymphocytes can be divided into subgroups based on cell surface markers as well as function. The B lymphocytes are the antibody factories of the immune response (secretors are termed plasma cells), and also function as antigen-presenting cells (APCs) for the T helper lymphocytes. This latter group can be considered the orchestrators of the specific response, and carry out this mission through secretion of various cytokines, soluble messengers of the immune response. This group can be subdivided further based on the direction in which the T helper cell pushes the response, and are designated by subtype numbers or descriptions: T_H1, T_H2, T_H17, and T regulatory lymphocytes. A group of T lymphocytes distinct from T helper lymphocytes is the cytotoxic T lymphocytes, the hired assassins. They specifically target cells that have been altered, such as by microbial invasion, and induce apoptosis in the target cell, in essence removing the microbial factory.

THE INNATE RESPONSE

The initial encounter of pathogen and host in most infections occurs on the mucosal or cutaneous surfaces. A variety of defensive mechanisms exist on these surfaces to protect the animal from infectious agents. The epithelial lining and the underlying connective tissue itself provide a barrier to penetration. On mucosal surfaces, mucus secretions serve to trap particles, making them easier to remove. In the respiratory and urogenital tracts, ciliated epithelia propel mucus-entrapped microbes. Additional physiologic barriers, such as the inhospitable pH of the gastric environment, are also protective against invading microorganisms. These barriers are effective at protecting the animal, and serve as a primary defense mechanism. Should these barriers be breached, additional nonspecific defensive measures exist to provide rapid and effective protection in the form of soluble mediators and cells.

A wide variety of cells, including those at epithelial surfaces, produce antimicrobial substances that act as important effectors of innate immunity. These compounds fall into 3 basic functional groups[2]: (1) digestive enzymes with degradative capabilities, (2) peptides that bind essential nutritive elements, and (3) peptides that disrupt microbial structures. These substances are produced by epithelial cells and cells of the inflammatory response, among others. They may be expressed constitutively or expression may be induced by tissue damage or infection. Their activity is broad in its spectrum, targeting viruses, bacteria, fungi, and parasites. Examples of these soluble components include the enzyme lysozyme, found in tears and mucosal secretions, which is able to cleave the peptidoglycan layer of bacterial cell walls; lactoferrin, which binds iron, preventing its use by invading pathogens in the mammary gland; and complement, an enzymatic protein cascade activated by immune complexes or various microbial structures, producing chemoattractants, inflammatory mediators, opsonins and a hole-punching complex capable of damaging membrane structures.

Although the innate immune response is not specific in terms of antigen recognition, many components do have pattern recognition. Microbial agents contain unique molecules not found in higher organisms, referred to as pathogen-associated molecular patterns (PAMPs). These include lipopolysaccharide (LPS) of gram-negative bacteria, peptidoglycan of gram-positive bacteria, flagellin, and even microbial nucleic acid structures.[3] The receptors for these molecules, referred to as pathogen recognition receptors (PRRs), may be soluble in plasma, present on cell surfaces, or expressed within the cellular cytoplasm. In a soluble form, this pattern recognition ability may reside in molecules such as complement and some enzymes, leading ultimately to destruction of the microbe. Recognition and binding of microbes by receptors present on the surfaces of various cell types lead to activation of intracellular signaling pathways, altering gene expression, and facilitating elimination of the pathogen by these cells.[4] Toll-like receptors (TLRs) are one of the best studied PRRs.[5] These structures are present on the cellular or endosomal membrane, and recognize viral, bacterial, and protozoal structures. Another group of PRRs, the nucleotide oligomerization domain-like (NOD-like) receptors, are cytosolic and sense intracellular microbes, including viral structures.[3]

The phagocytic cells, including macrophages, dendritic cells, and neutrophils, express a variety of these PRRs, allowing recognition of pathogens, and enhancing phagocytosis and destruction of the pathogen by these cells. When the physical barriers of the animal are penetrated, an inflammatory response ensues, and these cells are critical players in this response. Neutrophils are often the first cells on the scene, and migrate from the blood vessels to the affected tissue. They are efficient phagocytes, and possess oxidative and nonoxidative mechanisms for microbial destruction. The former uses toxic reactive radicals (oxygen and nitrogen) in the phagolysosome; the latter includes enzymes and antimicrobial peptides, such as defensins.[2] Monocytes/macrophages and dendritic cells also use these mechanisms for pathogen destruction. In addition, these cells secrete several inflammatory mediators, and are integral to the adaptive, specific response by serving as antigen presenters for the T helper lymphocytes (described later) and through secretion of several important cytokines such as interleukin (IL)-1. Dendritic cells in particular are critical to the adaptive immune response, presenting antigen to cytotoxic T lymphocytes as well as T helpers.

NK cells are lymphocytes, but differ from T and B lymphocytes in many ways. The chief difference is their lack of antigen-specific receptors generated by gene rearrangement. They are critical early defenders against intracellular pathogens, targeting and killing infected cells as well as altered or cancerous cells. Recognition of the altered cell by the NK cell is accomplished through cell surface molecules and results in induction of apoptosis in the affected cell. They are also important immunomodulators, secreting cytokines such as interferon gamma, and tumor necrosis factor-alpha.[6] Recently, NK cells have been shown to mount secondary heightened responses to antigens encountered previously, leading to speculation that these cells are the evolutionary bridge between innate and adaptive immunity.[7]

Additional granulocytic cells, eosinophils, basophils, and mast cells are important defenders against parasitic invaders, and use similar antipathogen strategies as described earlier. In addition, they secrete important inflammatory mediators such as histamine, bradykinin, and prostaglandin.

As alluded to previously, many of the cells also produce small secreted proteins, referred to as cytokines and chemokines, that mediate intercellular communication. After binding receptors on various cells by cytokines, signaling pathways are initiated and a wide array of effects are produced. Depending on the cytokine and the responding cell, these effects may include induction of cellular growth and/or differentiation, expression of certain proteins, enhancement of cellular functions such as phagocytosis, or enhanced killing of microorganisms.[1] Some cytokines act as chemoattractants for various white blood cells and are referred to as chemokines. An important group of cytokines that function in innate immunity is the interferon family. Interferons mediate a variety of biologic functions and function as immunomodulators, as well as an inducer of an antiviral state in cells.

The innate immunity is an essential defensive system, but several aspects influence the response pattern of specific immunity. One of the most important roles of the innate system for the adaptive response is in antigen presentation, and 1 of the most critical cell types involved is the dendritic cell (this will be covered in more detail following the discussion of effector functions).

While the innate response is an evolutionarily ancient defense system, one that is present in the animal before pathogen invasion and providing immediate protection, the adaptive immune response is a more recent evolutionary development, and is a more sophisticated system. It possesses tremendous diversity and exquisite specificity of recognition, and after it responds, it leaves an expanded population of memory cells (Kuby). These characteristics of adaptive immunity reside in the B and T lymphocytes.

ADAPTIVE IMMUNITY

The adaptive immune response exists to specifically recognize and eliminate a pathogen. As stated earlier, the major cell type involved, and the only one with the unique properties of specificity, diversity of recognition, and memory, is the lymphocyte. In contrast to other cells of the immune response, lymphocytes have the ability to distinguish countless distinctive structures and recognize small slight differences among them, and they exhibit immunologic memory. Unlike the innate response, the adaptive response takes time to develop, but it also improves as it develops.

LYMPHOCYTES

Lymphocytes are divided into distinct types based on phenotype and function, but share some common properties. They achieve their tremendous diversity of recognition by rearrangement of the gene segments encoding their antigen receptors during development. They maintain their tolerance to self through a rigid selection process that occurs on completion of this gene rearrangement and the resultant commitment to a specific antigen. Lymphocyte types vary in the precise mechanism of antigen recognition, as well as effector functions.

B lymphocytes develop in the bone marrow, and express immunoglobulins on their surface that function in antigen recognition and binding. The immunoglobulins, made up of 2 heavy and 2 light polypeptide chains, are all identical on each individual B cell surface. They recognize soluble or extracellular epitopes that are conformation dependent. After antigen encounter, the B lymphocyte proliferates and differentiates into plasma cells or memory cells. Plasma cells are terminally differentiated and secrete soluble antibody. Antibody binding to the target mediates several effector functions, discussed later. The biologic function is determined in part by the antibody isotype or class, which is determined by the heavy chain structure. Memory cells are long-lived, are more easily activated than naive cells, and produce a heightened, better response upon antigen encounter.

Unlike B lymphocytes, T lymphocytes leave the bone marrow and mature in the thymus. The antigen-binding receptor of T lymphocytes is referred to as the T cell receptor. Like B lymphocytes, the T cell receptor diversity is generated by gene rearrangement. Unlike B lymphocytes, the T cell receptor recognizes antigen only when it is bound to self MHC molecules. These latter molecules fall into 2 categories: class I which are expressed on all nucleated cells and display peptides produced and processed within the cell (endogenously produced), and class II which are expressed on APCs and display peptides from proteins that were endo- or phagocytosed by the APC (exogenously produced). T lymphocytes are further divided into 2 lineages based on differing functions and cell surface markers. Cytotoxic T lymphocytes (T_C) expressing CD8 cell marker recognize antigen displayed on MHC I (expressed on all cells), and function to induce apoptosis in the cell displaying nonself or foreign antigen. T helper lymphocytes (T_H) display a CD4 membrane glycoprotein and function in modulation of the immune response via secreted molecules (cytokines) and cell surface molecule expression. They recognize antigen displayed on MHC II expressed on APCs, including macrophages and DCs as well as B lymphocytes. The cytokines secreted by the T_H cells are critical to cell-mediated and humoral responses. The pattern of cytokine secretion in essence directs and modulates the immune response so that the appropriate effector functions are elicited; the functional classification of T_H lymphocytes is based on this secretion pattern. Thus, the T_H1 subset promotes a cell-mediated response; the T_H2 subset promotes a humoral response. Additional biotypes of T helper cells include T_H17, which secretes the cytokine IL-17 among others and enhances responses to extracellular bacteria, and the Tregs, which are critical for preventing immune-mediated damage.

THE ANTIGEN ENCOUNTER

In the adaptive immune response, the lymphocyte must encounter the antigen for which it is specific. This process is facilitated by secondary lymphoid tissues (as opposed to primary lymphoid tissue, bone marrow, and thymus). These tissue sites, such as lymph nodes and spleen, facilitate this encounter by filtering and concentrating antigen from extracellular fluid and blood. These tissues are rich in lymphocytes and APCs, including macrophages and DCs. Within these tissues, cells are motile, scanning for antigen[8] and sampling the environment. Antigen encounter combined with appropriate intercellular signals leads to activation, proliferation, and differentiation of the responding lymphocytes. Activation results in alteration of gene expression, allowing the lymphocyte to carry out its function; proliferation ensures sufficient numbers of lymphocytes with the same antigenic specificity are available; and differentiation produces effector cells for the current infection as well as memory cells for subsequent encounters.

The mechanisms for antigen recognition differ among T and B lymphocytes. B lymphocytes bind free antigen, either soluble or on a cellular surface. The epitopes bound may be any biochemical structure, although most have a protein component. These structures are unmodified and in their native state. T lymphocytes can only bind antigen presented in MHC structures. MHC molecules are codominantly expressed (ie, both maternal and paternal alleles) and are less stringent in peptide binding than the antigen receptors on lymphocytes. For this presentation by MHC to occur, the antigen must be processed. As stated earlier, MHC class I molecules are expressed on all nucleated cells. These structures bind peptides from proteins produced and processed within the cellular cytosol. In a normal cell, these are self peptides; but in cells infected with an intracellular pathogen, or altered cells (eg, tumor cells), some of the MHC I structures display nonself peptides, targeting the cell for destruction by cytotoxic T lymphocytes. APCs express MHC II for presentation to T helper lymphocytes. The professional APCs are macrophages, B lymphocytes, and DCs. Other cells, such as fibroblasts and vascular endothelial cells, can display MHC II under inflammatory conditions. The origin of the peptides in MHC II is exogenous material, taken up by endo- or phagocytosis and processed in the endosomal pathway. Expression of nonself peptides in these structures activates the T helper lymphocyte.[1]

Naive lymphocytes, regardless of type, require costimulatory signals in addition to the detection of the specific antigen. For the T helper lymphocyte, this signal is provided by cell surface molecule interactions with the APC. For B and cytotoxic T lymphocytes, this signal is provided primarily by cytokine secretion by the T helper lymphocyte. Binding of antigen in the absence of this costimulation leads to induction of anergy in the lymphocyte; this is an important mechanism in the maintenance of peripheral tolerance.[1]

Once antigen is recognized by the lymphocyte and the costimulatory signal is received, the lymphocyte proliferates, producing more cells with the same antigenic specificity. These cells differentiate into effector cells to deal with the current infection, or memory cells for future infections with the same pathogen. The latter cells are long-lived and require only the antigen encounter for activation; the costimulatory signal is not needed. Thus, memory cells are more easily activated providing a rapid response to subsequent infections with the same pathogen.

EFFECTOR FUNCTIONS

The effector function is the crucial end point of any specific immune response. The humoral and cell-mediated effector functions play different roles in battling infection. The humoral response, constituted by antibodies, mediates protection against extracellular pathogens. The cell-mediated response, which is made up of not only cytotoxic T lymphocytes but also neutrophils, macrophages, and NK cells, combats intracellular pathogens by eliminating the cell that harbors them. The T helper lymphocytes are critical to humoral and cell-mediated functions.

Humoral immunity, the effector function of B lymphocytes, involves antibody secretion. Antibody binding to an antigen mediates several biologic activities. Binding of a pathogen by antibody can effectively neutralize the pathogen; the coating by antibody of important pathogen molecules prevents the functioning of the latter. Thus, viral attachment and uncoating, bacterial colonization, and receptor binding by toxin are all inhibited by the presence of bound neutralizing antibody. Antibodies also share the ability to agglutinate or clump pathogens given that all have at least 2 antigen-binding sites. The antibody isotype most efficient at agglutination is IgM, with its 10 antigen-binding sites. This agglutination provides for easier removal of the pathogens. Antibody bound to antigen also opsonizes the antigen, flagging it for phagocytosis by cells with receptors for the constant region of the antibody (Fc receptor). Binding of antibody to antigen on cells, such as virus-infected cells, will flag the cell for destruction by cells with Fc receptors, including NK cells and macrophages, referred to as antibody-dependent cell-mediated cytotoxicity. This is most commonly mediated by IgG. IgA is secreted as a dimer across mucosal surfaces and mediates its activity in the lumen (eg, in the intestines). These activities include agglutination and neutralization. IgE binds stably to mast cells via receptors on the cell. Cross-linking of the mast cell–bound IgE by antigen initiates mast cell degranulation. Mast cells are commonly found in tissue surrounding mucosal surfaces and their secretory granules contain important inflammatory mediators. This defense mechanism is important for protection against parasites.

IgM and IgG bound to antigen will activate the complement cascade. This is perhaps the most important effector function of antibodies. This cascade of enzymatic reactions uses a collection of serum proteins, mediates several biologic effects and can be activated by various microbial structures alone, such as mannose residues on certain bacteria. A key consequence of complement activation is assembly of a membrane attack complex, which forms a large pore in the membrane of the pathogen leading to osmotic lysis of the target. By-products of the complement pathway also mediate important functions, including opsonization of the microbe or immune complex for phagocytes with complement receptors (eg, macrophages, neutrophils); neutralization and aggregation of microbes; degranulation of mast cells (anaphylatoxins); smooth muscle contraction and increased vascular permeability; and chemotaxis for various white blood cells.

The effector function of cytotoxic T lymphocytes (CTL) is the elimination of altered or infected cells. Through recognition of nonself peptides in MHC I and T helper lymphocyte costimulation, the CTL engages the target cell and induces apoptosis. Directional release of cytoplasmic granules containing perforins and granzymes, as well as expression of a transmembrane molecule, Fas ligand, trigger the apoptic process in the target cell.

The T helper lymphocyte effector function is primarily cytokine secretion. As stated earlier, the pattern of cytokines secreted by this cell directs the immune response and defines the T helper subset. For example, T_H1 lymphocyte secrete interferon-γ and tumor necrosis factor-β, which promote the cell-mediated response and antagonize the humoral response. T_H2 lymphocyte, on the other hand, secrete cytokines such as IL-4 and IL-5, which induce antibody class-switching from IgM to IgG and IgE, and support eosinophil activity, all of which enhance parasite elimination. T_H17 lymphocyte secrete cytokines such as IL-17 and IL-22, and are important in defense against extracellular bacteria, especially at mucosal surfaces. The balance amongst these cells determines the success of the immune response.

Recently, a new lineage of T helper lymphocytes has been identified, referred to as T regulatory lymphocytes (Tregs). These cells are important in moderating inflammation and maintaining peripheral tolerance.[9] In addition to the CD4 cell surface marker, these cells express CD25 surface marker, and an important transcription factor referred to as FoxP3. They produce inhibitory cytokines (IL-10, TGF-β, IL-35), affect the function of and induce apoptosis of effector lymphocytes, and modulate the function of DCs. Tregs disrupt lymphocyte activation and block lymphocyte differentiation and effector functions.[10] The balance between Treg and effector cell functions is important in preventing autoimmune disease and chronic inflammatory diseases.[9]

The directional development of the T helper lymphocytes seems to depend on the nature of the antigen, coreceptor signaling, and the cytokine environment. The DC plays a critical role in this development. Through recognition of pathogen-specific structures by PRRs, the DC develops into a form able to activate the appropriate immune response to eliminate the pathogen[11] by cytokine secretion and costimulatory molecules, which then activate T helper subset-specific genes.

DENDRITIC CELLS

Dendritic cells (DCs) are members of the innate arm of the immune system and are present in all peripheral tissues, but they als o play a critical role in the adaptive response. DCs are major APCs, providing important signals for the T lymphocytes with which they interact. They are phagocytic, functioning in antigen capture and processing using the same types of mechanisms for microbial destruction as macrophages and neutrophils. These include oxygen and nitrogen radicals, antimicrobial peptides, and proteolytic enzymes. However, unlike eosinophils and neutrophils, degradation is incomplete, reserving immunogenic peptides for association with major histocompatibility complex (MHC) molecules. DCs possess the ability to present exogenously derived antigen in either MHC I or II to cytotoxic or helper T lymphocytes, respectively.[1] They use PRRs (especially TLRs) to detect microbes leading to phagocytosis and activation of the DC. Different subpopulations of DCs selectively express different PRRs which in turn initiate different programs in response to the infecting pathogen (ie, humoral vs cell-mediated responses).[12] Activation following PRR recognition of a particular pathogen leads to increased expression of class II MHC as well as costimulatory molecules on the DC surface necessary for T helper lymphocyte activation. DCs thus serve as important mediators of the adaptive immune response, alerting the T helper lymphocyte to the presence of a pathogen, and insuring that the proper immune response is induced by directing T helper lymphocyte differentiation into the appropriate effector classes: T helper 1 responses for intracellular pathogens, T helper 2 responses for extracellular pathogens, particularly helminths, and T helper 17 responses for extracellular bacteria and fungi.[13]

DCs also present immunogenic peptides to cytotoxic T lymphocytes via MHC I and provide costimulatory signals for their activation.[12] Normally, peptides presented in MHC I are endogenously produced in the cytosol of the presenting cell. These intracellularly produced proteins are processed by the cytosolic proteasome, and the resultant peptides transported into the endoplasmic reticulum (ER) for association with MHC I. In the event of cellular invasion by a microbe such as a virus, some of the peptides presented in MHC I are microbial in origin. These foreign peptides in MHC I alert cytotoxic T lymphocytes to the "altered state" of the cell, making it a target for destruction by these cells. DCs possess the ability to partially degrade the phagocytosed protein (microbe) and transport the resultant pieces into the DC cytoplasm. The protein pieces are then further degraded by the cytosolic proteasome and the resultant peptides are transported into the ER for association with MHC I, and referred to as cross-presentation.[12] This allows activation of cytotoxic T lymphocytes by DC cells.

After phagocytosis and processing, the DC migrates from its site in the skin or mucosal surface to the underlying lymphatics where presentation to T lymphocytes occurs.[4] It is thought that based on the signals generated by the binding of pathogen by the various PRR subtypes expressed on the DC (eg, TLR4 recognition of bacterial LPS), particular cell surface molecules and cytokines are produced that induce the appropriate T lymphocyte response.[4]

Another important function of DCs is speculated to be their role in antagonizing the immunosuppressive function of T regulatory lymphocytes (Tregs). In response to activation by microbial sensing and phagocytosis, cytokines produced prevent Tregs from quelling the immune response by T helpers and cytotoxic T cells.[4]

TOLERANCE

Integral to an appropriate lymphocyte response is the ability to distinguish self from nonself. Several important mechanisms are used to maintain a tolerance to self.[1] Central tolerance refers to the screening process occurring during lymphocyte development in the bone marrow (B lymphocytes) or thymus (T lymphocytes). During this process, self-reactive lymphocytes are identified and deleted through apoptosis. Safety measures exist for self-reactive cells that escape this process, termed peripheral tolerance. The mechanisms for peripheral tolerance include induction of anergy (antigen encounter without the costimulatory signal), Tregs, and antigen sequestration from lymphocytes. DCs play important roles in induction of anergy through lack of costimulation of T lymphocytes and activation of Tregs, which function in silencing self-reactive T lymphocytes.[14] Failure of these mechanisms leads to autoimmune disease.

THE BIG PICTURE

So what does it all mean and how does it all work together to eliminate the invader? The inflammatory process may be localized or systemic, and even localized responses are often accompanied by systemic responses such as fever and stimulation of white blood cell production.

The inflammatory and immune response is initiated by tissue damage or infection, which is detected by white blood cell surveillance. Cellular damage leads to release of vasoactive and chemotactic factors, which in turn leads to increased vascular permeability and vasodilation at the site.[1] This allows leakage of soluble mediators at the site of injury/infection. The vascular endothelial cells in the region begin to express cellular adhesion molecules, facilitating extravasation of white blood cells at the site of inflammation. Invading pathogens are initially detected by white blood cells of the innate response using TLRs. Once activated by pathogen detection, some of these leukocytes will release mediators that function in recruitment of effector cells. Among these, chemokines are important chemoattractants of additional leukocytes. Other chemoattractants include complement breakdown products and microbial peptides. In response, leukocytes are able to migrate to the scene following the trail of chemotactic factors. Neutrophils are often first on the scene, but other granulocytes, as well as tissue macrophages and DCs are involved. Phagocytosis and microbial destruction follow the arrival of these cells to the site.

The invading pathogens and tissue damage may be dealt with by the innate response. In most cases, however, the antigen-specific response mediated by lymphocytes follows, and requires the innate immunity.[15] Free antigen (breakdown products, whole organisms, by-products, and so forth.) as well as the activated APCs will migrate to regional lymph nodes to interact with B and T lymphocytes. The interaction of APCs and lymphocytes promotes lymphocyte activation, proliferation, and differentiation into effector and memory cells within the lymphoid tissue. The nonspecific and specific immunity thus collaborate to eliminate the pathogen.

Lymphocyte effectors will migrate to the site of inflammation, whereas memory lymphocytes will preferentially recirculate to the site of initial antigen encounter and activation. This process is mediated by cell adhesion molecules, referred to as vascular addressins expressed on lymphocytes and vascular endothelial cells. Although the effector cells mediate pathogen elimination by the activities described earlier, the memory cells persist to provide protection against future infections with the same pathogen. Memory cells are long-lived lymphocytes of heightened reactivity, producing a rapid response of higher magnitude than that of naive lymphocytes.

The immune response is simple in its goal, but complex in its achievement of this goal. The response must be carefully regulated to avoid significantly damaging the host; immune-mediated tissue damage is an important consequence of inflammation and the pathogenesis of several diseases affecting animals. Lack of function in any component of this response, whether inherited or secondary to an extraneous factor, can potentially be life threatening. The complexity of the immune response makes therapeutic manipulation of this response challenging but promising. In addition, manipulation of this response prophylactically has been exploited to control many infectious diseases in veterinary medicine. These issues are discussed in more detail in other articles in this issue.

ACKNOWLEDGMENTS

The author thanks Misty Bailey for technical editing of the manuscript.

REFERENCES

1. Kindt TJ, Goldsby RA, Osborne BA. Immunology. New York: WH Freeman and Company; 2007.
2. Linde A, Ross CR, Davis EG, et al. Innate immunity and host defense peptides in veterinary medicine. J Vet Intern Med 2008;22:247–65.
3. Franchi L, Warner N, Viani K, et al. Function of Nod-like receptors in microbial recognition and host defense. Immunol Rev 2009;227:106–28.
4. Takeuchi O, Akira S. Innate immunity to virus infection. Immunol Rev 2009;227: 75–86.
5. Lee KH, Iwasaki A. Innate control of adaptive immunity: dendritic cells and beyond. Semin Immunol 2007;19:48–55.
6. Andoniou CE, Andrews DM, Degli-Esposti MA. Natural killer cells in viral infection: more than just killers. Immunol Rev 2006;214:239–50.
7. Sun JC, Lanier LL. Natural killer cells remember: an evolutionary bridge between innate and adaptive immunity? Eur J Immunol 2009;39:2059–64.
8. Batista FD, Harwood NE. The who, how and where of antigen presentation to B cells. Nat Rev Immunol 2009;9:15–27.
9. Vignali DAA, Collison LW, Workman CJ. How regulatory T cells work. Nat Rev Immunol 2008;8:523–32.
10. Sojka DK, Huang YH, Fowell DJ. Mechanisms of regulatory T-cell suppression – a diverse arsenal for a moving target. Immunology 2008;124:13–22.
11. Kaiko GE, Horvat JC, Beagley KW, et al. Immunological decision-making: how does the immune system decide to mount a helper T-cell response? Immunology 2007;123:326–38.
12. Savina A, Amigorena S. Phagocytosis and antigen presentation in dendritic cells. Immunol Rev 2007;219:143–56.
13. Palm NW, Medzhitov R. Pattern recognition receptors and control of adaptive immunity. Immunol Rev 2009;227:221–33.

14. Cools N, Ponsaerts P, Van Tendeloo VFI, et al. Balancing between immunity and tolerance: an interplay between dendritic cells, regulatory T cells, and effector T cells. J Leukoc Biol 2007;82:1365–74.
15. Saalmuller A. New understanding of immunological mechanisms. Vet Microbiol 2006;117:32–8.

Vaccines in Veterinary Medicine: A Brief Review of History and Technology

Scott McVey, DVM, PhD[a],*, Jishu Shi, DVM, PhD[b]

KEYWORDS

- Vaccine • Vaccine technology • Immunization
- Vaccination efficacy

The use of vaccines in veterinary medicine has progressed from an experimental adventure to a routine and relatively safe practice. The common and aggressive use of efficacious vaccines has been, in large part, responsible for control and eradication of several diseases. However, despite progress in research technologies, diagnostic capabilities, and manufacturing methods, there remain many infectious diseases for which no effective vaccines exist. Global availability, field compliance, effectiveness, and safety are also significant concerns. This review addresses the history, current practices, and potential future improvements of vaccine use in veterinary medicine.

THE HISTORY OF VACCINES IN MEDICINE: VARIOLATION, VACCINATION, AND IMMUNIZATION

The development of vaccines and vaccination programs has been evolving for centuries. The observation that persons that had recovered from smallpox infections were immune to reinfection has been recorded throughout history by several societies. Many Eastern cultures practiced different forms of variolation for several centuries.[1] By the sixteenth century the practice of variolation (inoculating partially attenuated variola virus to prevent smallpox) was common in Europe.[2] This practice originated more or less simultaneously with the practice of inoculating lambs with sheep pox. In the latter years of the eighteenth century, cross-protective properties of the vaccinia virus (cow pox) allowed for the more socially acceptable practice of "vaccination" to

[a] School of Veterinary Medicine and Biomedical Sciences, College of Agriculture and Natural Resources, Nebraska Veterinary Diagnostic Center, University of Nebraska-Lincoln, PO Box 830907, Lincoln, NE 68583-0907, USA
[b] Department of Anatomy and Physiology, College of Veterinary Medicine, 232 Coles Hall, Kansas State University, Manhattan, KS 66506, USA
* Corresponding author.
E-mail address: dmcvey2@unlnotes.unl.edu

Vet Clin Small Anim 40 (2010) 381–392
doi:10.1016/j.cvsm.2010.02.001
0195-5616/10/$ – see front matter © 2010 Elsevier Inc. All rights reserved.

become a routine component of medicine.[3] Problems with consistent potency, available supply, purity, and safety were common. Nevertheless, both the effectiveness and imperfections of vaccination lead to the eventual global eradication of smallpox, and was the inspiration for development of the products and programs for immunization against several diseases in humans and animals.

Louis Pasteur first used the term vaccine in 1881 for immunogens directed at other diseases besides smallpox. Pasteur directed many investigations that demonstrated the feasibility of attenuating or inactivating microbes. Studies with fowl cholera and anthrax led to the concepts of chemical inactivation as a means to reduce the virulence of microorganisms.[4,5] Studies with erysipelas and rabies explored serial passage in animals (lapinization or passage through rabbits) or other animal derived tissues as an alternative strategy to reduce or eliminate virulence.[6] Thus, the virulence of infectious microbes could be completely or partially reduced. These studies have led to the eventual successful control of anthrax and rabies in particular. The work of Salmon and Smith[7] (1886) clearly demonstrated that some microbes could be completely inactivated (killed). These developments eventually led to successful immunization programs against typhoid fever, tuberculosis, rinderpest, and foot and mouth disease (FMD). Attenuation and inactivation principles were extended to microbial toxins by the work of Gaston Ramon at the Pasteur Institute.[8] A tetanus toxoid was developed in 1924 through heat and formalin inactivation of the toxin to form an "anatoxin." Also, enhanced efficacy was provided by absorbing the toxoid to an aluminum hydroxide, providing an adjuvant effect. These process and formulation improvements were developed and refined in the early twentieth century, first through production of equine sera with antidiphtheria and antitetanus toxin-neutralizing antibody for prophylactic use. In the modern era of vaccine use, these same basic technologies are still the mainstays of vaccine production. However, new generations of recombinant, nucleic acid and subunit vaccines have become available. It is remarkable that the principles of developmental research, registration, and manufacture still follow the techniques of the grand heritage.

During the early years of the modern era of vaccine production, infected tissues were often used as a source of microbial antigens through grinding, inactivation (typically with formaldehyde solutions), and subsequent filtration or clarification. More often than not these vaccines were produced in regional research institutions. Industrialization of the processes began in the 1930s and 1940s when large-scale, controlled processes were used to produce FMD antigens in Germany by Waldmann and colleagues.[9] The development of first primary and subsequently clean cell lines occurred in the 1950s and 1960s. Development of high-volume roller bottle methods and later large-scale bioreactors has made possible the production of millions of doses of vaccines.[2] Further, production has been maintained in secure, closed systems, enhancing the security for the environment as well as the technical staff. In like manner, improvements in inactivation technologies (cyclized binary ethyleneimines), purification and concentration of antigens, storage of bulk antigens, improved aluminum gels, and oil suspension adjuvants in the formulation of polyvalent antigens have been critical achievements in the steady advancements in vaccinology.[2]

As these technical advances were employed in the industry, independent and collaborative efforts by numerous governmental authorities created regulatory frameworks that have established regulations and guidelines for registration of new biologicals as well as consistent manufacture of pure, safe, and potent vaccines. Under these regulations all released lots of vaccines are tested to ensure consistent formulation characteristics and potency (immunologic strength), safety, and purity (sterility and freedom from contamination with extraneous biologic agents). Development of

Good Manufacturing Practices guidelines and master seed and master cell stock concepts has further ensured consistent manufacture of vaccines that will provide consistent immunogenicity and efficacy. A veterinary clinician therefore may use with confidence any approved vaccine as recommended by the manufacturer to achieve the anticipated clinical outcome of protection.

VACCINES IN CLINICAL PRACTICE IN VETERINARY MEDICINE

As the vaccine manufacturing processes improved with regard to consistency of biologic activity, robustness, and efficiency, routine clinical use of vaccines became more practical and economical.[10] There is no doubt that widespread use of efficacious vaccines has been associated with the global eradication of smallpox in humans and the regional control of FMD and rabies. The routine use of processed immunoglobulins (usually in the form of processed horse serum) preceded the use of vaccines. Although passive protection by the immunoglobulins is still employed (particularly for rabies and tetanus post exposure prophylaxis), the advantages of active immunity (immunologic memory and reduced risk of infection) have significantly reduced the use of passive immunity.

In the mid-1950s, veterinarians were commonly using rabies vaccines of brain tissue origin in dogs. The principal biologic products used in practice at that time were rabies vaccines, "viabilized" canine distemper/hepatitis virus vaccine and antisera, hog cholera and erysipelas vaccines and antisera, leptospirosis bacterins, and clostridial toxoids (**Fig. 1**). As the development and manufacturing capacity increased with time, vaccination of companion animals expanded to include rabies for cats, feline herpesvirus, parvovirus in cats and dogs, and feline calicivirus. **Table 1** describes the types of vaccines currently available to companion animal practitioners in most regions of the world[11–14] (http://www.aphis.usda.gov/animal_health/vet_biologics/vb_licensed_products.shtml) These vaccines include very traditional inactivated antigen formulations, multiple attenuated agents, and new technologies such as pox-vectored vaccines, defined subunit vaccines, and nucleic acid vaccines (see **Table 1**). The term vaccine is now used to describe many therapeutic or prophylactic formulations and products that stimulate active immunity in the vaccinated animal. This discussion focuses on vaccinations associated with infectious diseases.

Routine clinical use of these vaccines usually includes immunization of puppies and kittens at approximately 3-week intervals after maternal-derived antibody decreases to noninterfering titers. These immunization series are usually administered between the fourth and 16th weeks of life.[12,14] Puppies and kittens associated with unusual risk may be vaccinated at younger ages or at more frequent intervals. Rabies vaccination is usually first given at 4 months of age.[14] It is a common and efficacious practice to provide booster doses at 1 year of age for most vaccines.[14] These immunization practices will provide a solid duration of immunity of at least 5 to 7 years and longer in some cases. General recommendations (World Small Animal Veterinary Association) are to vaccinate every third year after the initial immunization series, and these recommendations are consistent with product label guidelines.[12] These initial immunization guidelines are derived from the initial registration immunogenicity and efficacy studies for any individual vaccine product. The efficacy studies define the minimum immunologic strength for the vaccine (the potency that must be present when the vaccine lot goes out of date). These same types of studies also define the minimum age of animals that can be successfully immunized as well as the specifics of the initial and booster immunization regimens (part 9, Code of Federal Regulations). It has

A

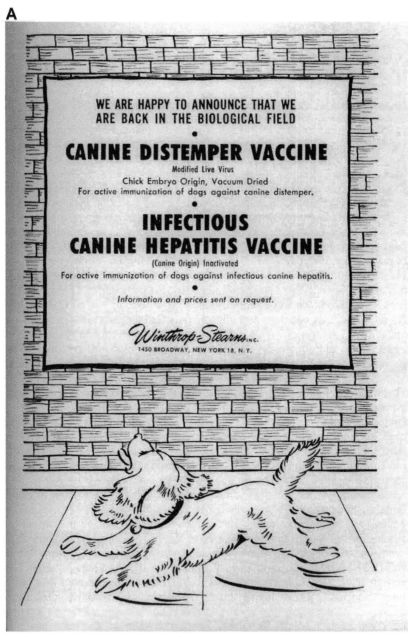

Fig. 1. (*A*, *B*) Examples of biologicals available in as published in the Journal of the American Veterinary Medical Association in 1955.

become very clear that many vaccines provide effective and long-term immunity for an extended period of time.[11] Over the past 3 decades, cumulative evidence for extended duration of immunity has been provided to support the 3-year booster intervals for most vaccines in dogs and cats. However, as described in **Table 1**, the relative efficacy of some vaccines is less than ideal.

B

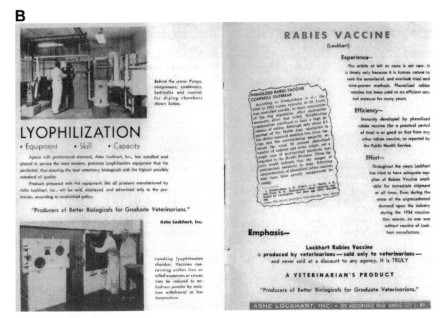

Fig. 1. (*continued*)

VACCINE EFFICACY AND EFFECTIVENESS

"Ideal" immunity would be not only protection from clinical disease (morbidity and mortality) but also blocking the infection/replication/spread or progression of infectious agents. Some vaccines do achieve this degree of protection. Some, however, may only reduce morbidity and/or mortality without generating a sterilizing immunity. Based on clinical and microbiological outcomes of an efficacy study challenge of immunity, various degrees of protection may be achieved and therefore claimed. The United States Department of Agriculture (USDA) has recognized these differences through a hierarchy of efficacy claims that may be allowed for a vaccine based on the outcomes of efficacy studies (**Box 1**).

The degree of efficacy and claim structures are usually derived from direct investigations of efficacy and challenge of immunity studies in their respective host animal species. Vaccinated and nonvaccinated animals are challenged with fully virulent organisms, and the degree of protection (efficacy) is determined under controlled settings. These classic studies are adequate to establish the efficacy of the vaccine but are not always sufficient to estimate the field effectiveness of a vaccine, or, in other words, the ability of a vaccine to control disease in the field. Effective control of infectious disease should result in reduced incidence and prevalence.[15,16] This would be true of not only clinical disease but also of infection and spread of the infectious agent. It is very clear that use of efficacious products has reduced incidence of rabies, particularly in dogs. Immunization of dogs has reduced the incidence of canine rabies to essentially nil in the United States and western Europe.[17] The rabies immunization programs in these countries have been so effective that most manufacturers of rabies vaccine for dogs and cats have switched to master seeds from canine street strains of virus to other types of terrestrial rabies (bat strains, for instance) to protect from the most significant current threats in these regions.

Table 1
Vaccines available for veterinary use

Antigen	Strain	Type	Relative Efficacy
Canine distemper virus	Rockborn, Snyder Hill, Oondersport, canary pox	MLV/recombinant nonreplicating in canary pox	High
Canine adenovirus	Type 1 (historical) Type 2	MLV	High
Canine parvovirus	Type 1 (historical) Type 2	MLV Inactivated	High, although some antigenic variation may exist
Rabies virus (canine and feline)	Bat strain (historical canine street strain virus)	Inactivated recombinant nonreplicating in canary pox (feline)	High
Feline panleukopenia virus	Feline origin	MLV and inactivated	High
Feline herpesvirus	Feline origin	MLV	Good for clinical disease
Feline calicivirus	Multiple serotypes	MLV	Moderate, strain gaps
Canine coronavirus	Canine origin	MLV and inactivated	Moderate, questionable DOI
Canine parainfluenza	Canine origin	MLV	Moderate
Bordetella bronchiseptica (canine and feline)	Canine origin	Bacterin and inactivated	Questionable
Leptospirosis bacterins, multiple serotypes	Canine origin	Inactivated	Moderate to good
Borrelia burgdorferi	Canine origin	Inactivated bacterin and OspA recombinant vaccine	Moderate

Abbreviations: DOI, duration of immunity; MLV, modified live virus.

Data from Day MJ, Horzinek MC, Schultz RD. Guidelines for the vaccination of dogs and cats. Compiled by the Vaccination Guidelines Group (VGG) of the World Small Animal Veterinary Association (WSAVA). J Small Anim Pract 2007;48:528–41; and Patel JR, Heldens JG. Review of companion animal viral diseases and immunoprophylaxis. Vaccine 2009;27:491–504.

Vaccination has also greatly reduced the incidence of canine distemper, canine parvovirus, infectious canine hepatitis, feline panleukopenia, and feline herpes virus infections as well as other diseases.[13] When these diseases do occur, there are usually issues with vaccine dose compliance, vaccination of sick or immunocompromised animals, exposure to wildlife, or problems associated with vaccine handling and/or administration. In situations where vaccines do not provide prevention of infection, concurrent infections may exist and vaccine failures are therefore more common. There are often issues with type-specific protections. For instance, it is not clear that available vaccines can protect cats against all types of calicivirus infections. Continual vigilance is required to ensure continued protection of animals in the face of potential newly evolving and emerging pathogens (eg, rabies and other lyssaviruses, canine distemper and parvoviruses, and feline calicivirus).

Box 1
Efficacy claims on USDA-regulated biologic products

Veterinary Services Memorandum NO. 800.202 (USDA-APHIS-CVB)

Subject: General Licensing Considerations: Efficacy Studies

To: Biologics Licensees, Permittees, and Applicants

4.2 *Label claims.*

- 4.2.1 *Prevention of infection.* A claim that it is intended to prevent infection may be made only for products able to prevent all colonization or replication of the challenge organism in vaccinated and challenged animals. If such a conclusion is supported with a very high degree of confidence by convincing data, a label statement such as "for the prevention of infection with [specific microorganism]" may be used.

- 4.2.2 *Prevention of disease.* A claim that it is intended to prevent disease may be made only for products shown to be highly effective in preventing clinical disease in vaccinated and challenged animals. The entire 95% interval estimate of efficacy must be at least 80%. If so, a label statement such as "for the prevention of disease due to [specific microorganism]" may be used.

- 4.2.3 *Aid in disease prevention.* A claim that it is intended to aid in disease prevention may be made for products shown to prevent disease in vaccinated and challenged animals by a clinically significant amount which may be less than that required to support a claim of disease prevention (section 4.2.2). If so, a label statement such as "as an aid in the prevention of disease due to [specific microorganism]" may be used.

- 4.2.4 *Aid in disease control.* A claim that it is intended to aid in disease control may be made for products which have been shown to alleviate disease severity, reduce disease duration, or delay disease onset. If so, a label statement such as "as an aid in the control of disease due to [specific microorganism]" or a similar one stating the product's particular action may be used.

- 4.2.5 *Other claims.* Products with beneficial effects other than direct disease control, such as the control of infectiousness through the reduction of pathogen shedding, may make such claims if the size of the effect is clinically significant and well supported by the data.

HOW DO VACCINES WORK?

The vaccines used in veterinary medicine generally fall into 1 of 3 categories: inactivated vaccines (in which antigens are typically combined with adjuvants); attenuated, live vaccines; and recombinant technology vaccines, which may include subunit antigens or genetically engineered organisms. In practice, combination and multivalent vaccines may employ all 3 approaches. All of these technologies have been used successfully, and each approach has inherent advantages and disadvantages. The protective mechanisms associated with vaccines are also becoming clearer.

Historically, the most common correlate of immunity to derive from vaccination has been measurements of antibody responses.[18,19] Antibodies have several functions including facilitating opsonization, complement-mediated cellular lysis, neutralization-blocking adherence or replication, and facilitating cytotoxic cells. However, mature, well-differentiated immune responses are the consequence of cumulative, regulated interactions between phagocytic cells, antigen-presenting cells, and both B and T lymphocytes. Therefore, a well-differentiated antibody response with isotype switching, affinity maturation to high avidity, and memory requires some effective initial stimulation involving dendritic cells and expansion of regulatory T lymphocytes (likely CD4+) and B lymphocytes. This stimulation phase is followed by a phase of differentiation into effector/memory T cells, B cells, and plasma cells.

With respect to the nature of pathogenesis of many infectious agents, the adaptive immune response to the vaccine often blocks or interferes with a specific segment of the infection process. For instance, antibody-mediated neutralization of rabies virus in extracellular spaces inhibits transmission to neurons and subsequent axonal progression of the virus to the central nervous system. In this case the presence of preformed, neutralizing antibody is critical for protection. A summary of protective characteristics of the immune responses to vaccines (as potential correlates of protection and disease prevention) is provided in **Table 2**. Although antibody responses are good correlates of protection, they do not always reflect all available protective mechanisms provided by a well-differentiated immune response. In some cases, other correlates are available. It is clear that the presence of neutralizing, vaccine-derived antibody will reduce mucosal virus replication, virus shedding, and viremia in kittens vaccinated with modified live feline herpes vaccines.[20–22] However, regulated CD4+ and CD8+ cellular responses are required to control tissue damage and reactivation of disease.[23] In this case, antibody may be a protective correlate of infection while cellular immunity is a protective correlate of disease. The ability of modified live vaccines to generate a very rapid onset of cytokines and interferons (and rapid antigen focusing in dendritic

Table 2
Potential adaptive mechanisms of protection/correlates of immunity

Correlate of Protection	Description	Prevent Infection?	Vaccine Characteristics
Neutralizing antibody (viral or bacterial, adhesion factors, toxins)	IgG, matching field strains or outbreak strains	Yes, potentially	MLV or inactivated, toxoids, nonreplicating viruses and particles
Nonneutralizing antibody (virus)	IgG, potentially interfering	Questionable	MLV or inactivated, any formulation
Nonneutralizing antibody (bacteria)	IgM or IgG, somatic antigens, opsonizing and complement-mediated clearance	Yes	Bacterins or attenuated vaccines
Mucosal surface protection	IgA, viral or bacterial, adhesion factors, toxins	Yes, if infection occurs at mucosal surface, may limit infection and shedding	Attenuated vaccines, especially in intranasal or oral
Virus-specific, cytotoxic T cells	CD8+ T cells, MHC-restricted killing of infected cells	Yes, limit infection spread and pathology by destruction of infected cells	Primarily attenuated vaccines, but newer formulations with novel adjuvants
T-helper cells	CD4+ T cells	Help differentiate antibody- and cell-mediated responses, essential for memory	Attenuated and inactivated formulations with appropriate adjuvants

Data from Rimmelzwaan GF, McElhaney JE. Correlates of protection: novel generations of influenza vaccines. Vaccine 2008;26 Suppl 4:D41–4.

cells in lymphoid tissues) is associated with a rapid onset of protection, even though antibody responses may not be detectable in serum for up to 2 weeks.[20–22] Therefore, the early response of multiple cytokines and concurrent activation of the innate immune system may serve as early correlates of protection.

There are also documented cases in which functional immunity outlasts detectable circulating antibody; this is true with many herpesvirus infections. However, the presence of detectable neutralizing serum antibody is correlated with protection against recrudescent disease.[23] In situations where vaccinated animals may be exposed to heterotypic viruses or bacteria, the presence of immune CD4+ T cells specific to conserved antigens may be very important for protection.[24] It is possible that the effective mechanisms for development of protection associated with a vaccine may be specific to the nature of the disease and infectious process. Recent studies have provided important information regarding this phenomenon. A common hypothesis is that vaccine-induced immunity should reflect convalescent immunity following natural infection. For example, It is known that recovery from primary poxvirus infections requires robust cytokine responses, natural killer cells, and antibodies as well as T helper (CD4) and cytotoxic T (CD8) lymphocyte effector functions.[25] However, recovery from a secondary infection requires only T- and B-lymphocyte interaction and an anamnestic antibody response. Again, neutralizing antibody will reduce infection, viremia, and spread of a virus (and may do so to the extent of blocking infection) while T-cell–mediated responses will allow survival and recovery. It seems clear that balanced antibody and cellular responses are necessary for complete protection from infection and disease as well as spread to other animals.

It should be mentioned that not all antigen-binding antibodies are protective. In some cases, such as with influenza virus, canine distemper virus, and herpesvirus vaccines, nonneutralizing antibody may be produced that does not contribute to the blocking of infection or enhancing clearance of the infectious agent.[24,26] For this reason, correlates or surrogates of protection should be linked to protective mechanisms; this can be done through retrospective analysis of data from efficacy and immunogenicity studies or through associational studies in immune populations (such as with primary vaccinates in an efficacy study).

FUTURE DEVELOPMENTS IN VACCINE TECHNOLOGY

Veterinary vaccinology has realized significant successes that have affected human and animal well-being, and the ability to coexist. The virtual elimination of canine rabies in North America and western Europe has indirectly led to human-animal bonding at a very intimate level that was not feasible when canine rabies was relatively common. However, there remain many diseases for which no efficacious or effective vaccine exists. Many parasitic diseases as well as diseases of a chronic, intracellular nature are not covered by any available vaccine. In some cases safety profiles or efficacy characteristics of existing vaccines are not acceptable. Fortunately, there are promising technologies that may close the technical gaps for prevention of these challenging diseases.

The processes of absorption of antigens such as chemically inactivated toxoids or viruses to aluminum gels, or the creation of water-in-oil emulsions of antigen particles have been the principal methods used for veterinary vaccine formulations. In some cases compounds such as crude or purified saponins (Quil A), squalenes, or pluronic block copolymers have been added to enhance immune stimulation.[27,28] Although these practices have been successful, newer technologies such as CpG DNA, defense peptides, imidazoquinolones, and polyphosphazenes may enhance both safety and efficacy.[28,29] Further, additional cholesterol and phospholipids may be combined with antigens and saponins to create immunostimulating complexes (ISCOMS) particles. Similar adjuvant particles can be generated with no antigen (ISCOMATRIX) that can be admixed directly with antigen suspensions. These advanced formulations may be used to provide very efficient adjuvants to in turn allow development of microvolume formulations as well as transdermal applications. Also, as better understanding of immune genotypes and phenotypes in animal populations emerges, individualized formulations of vaccines may be developed and produced that may enhance safety and efficacy.[30]

Proteomic technologies may very well provide methods to identify antigen subsets from among complex organisms and infectious agents such as bacteria and protozoa. These organisms contain large, complex genomes. Antigen expression is often dependent on growth conditions, and the medium may be very complex.[31] These conditions are difficult to reproduce and regulate in vitro. The combination of transcriptional and proteomic analysis may provide a means to identify key antigens associated with tissue or cellular persistence and potential virulence. Such analyses could provide means to simplify vaccine formulations to include only protective antigens and reduce the presence of nonprotective, potentially interfering bacterial proteins. Not only would this potentially improve efficacy, but it could also improve safety profiles by reducing the antigenic mass in a vaccine dose.

The continued use of alternative expression systems has many potential advantages. Transgenic expression of protein antigens and plant-based systems may provide access to oral vaccines as well as enhanced stability of antigens.[32] Expression of antigens in avirulent viruses, bacteria, and yeast and insect cells may provide both manufacturing and user safety by eliminating the need to use a virulent or partially virulent microbe to provide immunity.[33] Further development of nucleic acid vaccines may provide even greater formulation simplicity and biosecurity. Viral particles such as capsids from avirulent viruses may serve as building blocks to deliver nucleic acids, protein subunit antigens, and microadjuvants directly to secondary lymphoid tissue. Not only would these biologically engineered vaccines provide targeted immunity and eliminate the need to work with dangerous microbes, they very likely would reduce the time required for the onset of immunity, with excellent safety characteristics.

One of the most pressing problems associated with manufacturing vaccines is the requirement to rapidly modify antigen formulations as new diseases emerge or as older pathogens mutate and reemerge. Transcriptomics and proteomics combined with established recombinant or synthetic approaches could potentially provide antigens that could be rapidly formulated with approved new-generation adjuvants to produce novel and efficacious vaccines.[31] These technologies are commonplace in experimental laboratories. Using combinations of proteomics, reverse genetics, recombinant or molecular syntheses, and stable, consistent adjuvant platforms will allow development of "first line of defense" vaccines for a rapidly emerging disease in a short time. Such a use-inspired approach to vaccines would allow the use of assembly-line techniques to manufacture vaccines. As new antigens are required they could be selected, evaluated, and produced in a short period of time, and inserted directly into an established production system. This process would greatly reduce the time required for exploratory research and early development. Classic development cycles may require 5 to 7 years and sometimes may require even longer times for unusual or new types of pathogenic microbes. A reduction of the development time by 30% to 80% may be achievable using newer research and development technologies.

It is clear that new methods to assess efficacy and definitive, direct correlates of immunity also need to be identified. It is also clear that use of the many new technical achievements and discoveries will require advances in the regulatory framework to ensure more efficient but adequate evaluation of new biologicals. Vaccine development faces many technical, political, and ethical challenges.[34] The history of vaccine research and development as well as the continued use of immunization as the principal method to prevent infectious disease predict that the innovative experimental procedures of today will lead to common clinical applications tomorrow.

REFERENCES

1. Needham J. China and the origins of immunology. East Horiz 1980;19:6–12.
2. Lombard M, Pastoret PP, Moulin AM. A brief history of vaccines and vaccination. Rev Sci Tech 2007;26:29–48.
3. Jenner E. An inquiry into the causes and effects of the variolae vaccinae, a disease discovered in some of the western counties of England. Particularly Gloucestershire, and known by the name of The Cow Pox. London: Samson Low; 1798. p. 75.
4. Pasteur L. De l'atttenuation du virus du cholera des poules. Comptes rendus de l'Academie des Sciences 1880;91:673–80 [in French].
5. Pasteur L, Chamberland C, Roux E. Compte rendu sommaire des experiences faites a Pouilly-le Fort, pres Melun, sur la vaccination charbonneuse. Comptes rendus de l'Academie des Sciences 1881;92:1378–83 [in French].
6. Pasteur L. Method pour prevenir la rage apres morsure. Comptes rendus de l'Academie des Sciences 1885;101:765–73 [in French].
7. Salmon DE, Smith T. On a new method of producing immunity from contagious diseases. American Veterinary Review 1886;10:63–9.
8. Ramon G. Sur la toxine et l'anatoxine diphtheriques. Pouvir floculant et proprietes immunoantes. Ann Inst Pasteur 1924;38:1–10 [in French].
9. Waldmann D, Kobe K, Pyl G. Die aktive immunisierung des Rindes gegen Maul und Klauenseuche. Orig. Zentralbl Bakteriol 1937;401 [in German]
10. Horzinek MC, Thiry E. Vaccines and vaccination: the principles and the polemics. J Feline Med Surg 2009;11:530–7.
11. Schultz RD. Duration of immunity for canine and feline vaccines: a review. Vet Microbiol 2006;117:75–9.
12. Day MJ, Horzinek MC, Schultz RD. Guidelines for the vaccination of dogs and cats. Compiled by the Vaccination Guidelines Group (VGG) of the World Small Animal Veterinary Association (WSAVA). J Small Anim Pract 2007;48:528–41.
13. Patel JR, Heldens JG. Review of companion animal viral diseases and immunoprophylaxis. Vaccine 2009;27:491–504.
14. Davis-Wurzler GM. Current vaccination strategies in puppies and kittens. Vet Clin North Am Food Anim Pract 2006;36:607–40, vii.
15. Warrell MJ. Emerging aspects of rabies infection: with a special emphasis on children. Curr Opin Infect Dis 2008;21:251–7.
16. Zadoks RN, Schukken YH. Use of molecular epidemiology in veterinary practice. Vet Clin North Am Food Anim Pract 2006;22:229–61.
17. Rupprecht CE, Hanlon CA, Hemachudha T. Rabies re-examined. Lancet Infect Dis 2002;2:327–43.
18. Plotkin SA. Vaccines: correlates of vaccine-induced immunity: an official publication of the Infectious Diseases Society of America. Clin Infect Dis 2008;47:401–9.

19. Boni MF. Vaccination and antigenic drift in influenza. Vaccine 2008;26(Suppl 3): C8–14.
20. Jas D, Aeberlé C, Lacombe V, et al. Onset of immunity in kittens after vaccination with a non-adjuvanted vaccine against feline panleucopenia, feline calicivirus and feline herpesvirus. Vet J 2009;182:86–93.
21. Lappin MR, Veir J, Hawley J. Feline panleukopenia virus, feline herpesvirus-1, and feline calicivirus antibody responses in seronegative specific pathogen-free cats after a single administration of two different modified live FVRCP vaccines. J Feline Med Surg 2009;11:159–62.
22. Tham KM, Studdert MJ. Antibody and cell-mediated immune responses to feline herpesvirus 1 following inactivated vaccine and challenge. Zentralbl Veterinarmed B 1987;34:585–97.
23. Scott FW, Geissinger CM. Long-term immunity in cats vaccinated with an inactivated trivalent vaccine. Am J Vet Res 1999;60:652–8.
24. Rimmelzwaan GF, McElhaney JE. Correlates of protection: novel generations of influenza vaccines. Vaccine 2008;26(Suppl 4):D41–4.
25. Panchanathan V, Chaudhri G, Karupiah G. Correlates of protective immunity in poxvirus infection: where does antibody stand? Immunol Cell Biol 2008;86:80–6.
26. Vecht U, Wisselink HJ, Jellema ML, et al. Identification of two proteins associated with virulence of Streptococcus suis type 2. Infect Immun 1991;59:3156–62.
27. Garlapati S, Facci M, Polewicz M, et al. Strategies to link innate and adaptive immunity when designing vaccine adjuvants. Vet Immunol Immunopathol 2009; 128:184–91.
28. Mutwiri G, Gerdts V, Lopez M, et al. Innate immunity and new adjuvants. Rev Sci Tech 2007;26:147–56.
29. Schijns VE, Degen WG. Vaccine immunopotentiators of the future. Clin Pharmacol Ther 2007;82:750–5.
30. Poland GA, Ovsyannikova IG, Jacobson RM. Personalized vaccines: the emerging field of vaccinomics. Expert Opin Biol Ther 2008;8:1659–67.
31. Jagusztyn-Krynicka EK, Dadlez M, Grabowska A, et al. Proteomic technology in the design of new effective antibacterial vaccines. Expert Rev Proteomics 2009;6: 315–30.
32. Tacket CO. Plant-based oral vaccines: results of human trials. Curr Top Microbiol Immunol 2009;332:103–17.
33. Bae K, Choi J, Jang Y, et al. Innovative vaccine production technologies: the evolution and value of vaccine production technologies. Arch Pharm Res 2009; 32:465–80.
34. Poland GA, Jacobson RM, Ovsyannikova IG. Trends affecting the future of vaccine development and delivery: the role of demographics, regulatory science, the anti-vaccine movement, and vaccinomics. Vaccine 2009;27:3240–4.

Adverse Vaccinal Events in Dogs and Cats

George E. Moore, DVM, MS, PhD*, Harm HogenEsch, DVM, PhD

KEYWORDS

• Vaccinal events • Causality • Reactions
• Cytokines • Immunogenicity

Vaccines are the most successful application of immunologic principles to animal and human health, dramatically reducing the mortality and morbidity of infectious diseases. This disease reduction has also decreased public awareness of infectious disease risk and, perhaps paradoxically, shifted current public focus to the safety of vaccines. The immunologic stimulation from vaccines that provides protection sometimes produces undesired side effects, decreasing public confidence in and compliance with vaccination recommendations.

Undesired biologic events can occur for a myriad of reasons, and cause and effect may be difficult to determine in events following vaccination. Bradford-Hill in 1965 proposed a set of criteria as supporting evidence that an association is cause and effect.[1] Of these criteria, temporality (the cause precedes the effect) and/or biologic plausibility often provide strong support for cause and effect, particularly when the adverse events occur within a few minutes or a few hours after vaccination. Because of the uncommon or rare occurrence of some adverse events, however, causal support may be quite weak for other important criteria such as strength (large relative risk), consistency (repeatedly observed), or specificity (one cause leads to one effect). In general, the association of vaccination with development of disease is based upon a close temporal relationship *and* additional supportive epidemiological evidence. Defining an association as causal is further complicated by the occurrence of similar immune-mediated diseases in unvaccinated individuals or individuals without a history of recent vaccination.

Assessment of suspected adverse events is markedly hindered by current reporting systems. Reporting is voluntary; veterinarians or owners may contact either the manufacturer or the United States Department of Agriculture (USDA) Center for Veterinary Biologics (CVB), which has regulatory overwatch of animal vaccines: http://www.aphis.usda.gov/animal_health/vet_biologics/. Although servicing the total population, spontaneous systems are disadvantaged in that underreporting is

Department of Comparative Pathobiology, School of Veterinary Medicine, Purdue University, 725 Harrison Street, West Lafayette, IN 47907, USA
* Corresponding author.
E-mail address: gemoore@purdue.edu

Vet Clin Small Anim 40 (2010) 393–407
doi:10.1016/j.cvsm.2010.02.002
0195-5616/10/$ – see front matter

common and denominator data are lacking.[2–4] Reports are not screened out, and reporting rates may be influenced by external pressures, for example, the media. Although more vaccines are used overall in large animals than in small, most adverse events reported to CVB are in dogs and cats.[4] To improve vaccine safety studies, other large population databases can be useful in providing selected denominator data and determining background incidence rates.[5,6] Some adverse vaccinal effects are more commonly seen in certain breeds of dogs as discussed in this article, suggesting a genetic predisposition for these effects. This idea is supported by recent studies in human populations immunized against smallpox in which adverse reactions were associated with several gene variants.[7,8]

Adverse vaccinal events are generally uncommon because of good manufacturing practices and procedures used by the biologics industry. Inadvertent pathogen/pyrogen contamination of a vaccine or failure to sufficiently inactivate a live pathogen used for a vaccine can clearly produce an undesired, even lethal, effect. This article focuses on undesirable immune responses from vaccination of presumably healthy pets but does not discuss clinical manifestations of diseases for which the vaccine should have provided protection, for example, vaccine-induced distemper or rabies. Disease initiation by modified live virus or inadequately attenuated biologicals may occur in almost any animal that is sufficiently immunocompromised.

INNATE IMMUNE RESPONSES TO VACCINES

Vaccines induce both innate and adaptive immune responses, with the latter providing protection from natural disease exposure by immunologic memory. The innate response provides a rapid and necessary, but nonspecific, first line of defense while providing stimulation of the immune system for subsequent development of specific adaptive immune responses. The quality and quantity of immune memory is largely determined by the magnitude and complexity of innate immune signals that imprint the acquired immune response.[9,10]

The innate immune response can be triggered by tissue damage, that is, tissue disruption caused by injection of a vaccine, and by pathogen-associated molecular patterns (PAMPs), which are conserved molecular patterns produced by pathogens but not by the host organism.[11] PAMPs are detected in the host by different pattern-recognition receptors (PRRs), such as toll-like receptors (TLRs), which are expressed on a wide variety of immune cells, for example, neutrophils, macrophages, dendritic cells, natural killer (NK) cells, and B cells, as well as some nonimmune cells such as epithelial and endothelial cells.[12] Engagement of PRRs leads to the activation and secretion of cytokines and chemokines, in addition to the maturation and migration of antigen-presenting cells. In tandem, this creates an inflammatory environment that leads to the establishment of the adaptive immune response.[13,14]

Although an adaptive immune response is required for the primary (label) vaccine antigen (and is the goal of vaccination), other vaccine components serve as immune potentiators to stimulate the innate immune system. These components can include bacterial products, toxins, lipids, nucleic acids, peptidoglycans, peptides, carbohydrates, hormones, or other small molecules. Some components, commonly termed adjuvants, are purposefully added to vaccine formulations to enhance immunogenicity, but many components serve a similar role in vivo. Vaccine delivery systems, such as liposomes, emulsions, and microparticles, can also improve the adaptive response by concentrating and colocalizing antigens and immune potentiators.[13]

The cytokines and chemokines released by cells after activation of PRRs are mediators of inflammation, and include tumor necrosis factor α (TNF-α), interleukins (ILs), histamine, serotonin, complement, and leukotrienes. Different amounts of each mediator can be evoked from ligands triggering different PRRs, creating different cytokine "profiles". Cytokine profiles differ not only with the triggering mechanism but likely also between and within host species. Thus, the severity and type of localized inflammatory reactions to vaccines varies depending on the vaccine composition, route of administration, genetic makeup, and other individual differences among the recipients and species.

An adequate innate immune response that guides an appropriate adaptive response is desired, but clinically obvious nonspecific innate responses such as fever, lethargy, swelling, and soreness are not preferred sequelae to vaccination. Although a normal toxicity from vaccination might be expected, it is still preferential to minimize this toxicity for the patient and client's sake. Because various vaccine components can serve as immune potentiators, it is not surprising that a greater exposure (volume of vaccine received per kg body weight) increases the risk of a clinical focal or systemic reaction.[5,15,16] Minimizing the number of vaccines administered in a single office visit can reduce the risk of these undesired vaccine-associated adverse events.

Prevaccination prevention of such adverse events through administration of nonsteroidal antiinflammatory drugs (NSAIDs), for example, acetaminophen or aspirin, is sometimes used in human medicine, but inhibition of cyclooxygenase 2 (COX-2) may attenuate antibody response.[17] Known toxicities of these NSAIDs in cats in particular and in dogs, coupled with challenges in proper dose administration, has generally precluded their similar use in veterinary medicine.

HYPERSENSITIVITY REACTIONS
Type I

Immediate hypersensitivity (type I) produces IgE-mediated allergic reactions with degranulation of mast cells and basophils. Allergens are proteins, generally with a molecular weight between 10 and 40 kDa, which in low doses induce differentiation of T_H cells into T_H2 cells producing IL-4 and IL-5. IL-4 regulates the production of IgE and also enhances the growth of T_H2 cells. IgE is typically found in very low concentrations in serum because of its low production, short half-life (approximately 2 days), and sequestration on mast cells and basophils. IgE binds both high-affinity and low-affinity IgE receptors, and high-affinity IgE receptors are typically found only on mast cells and basophils. Mast cells and basophils are the primary histamine-holding cells in the body. When a relevant allergen cross-links 2 specific IgE molecules, signal transduction with calcium influx causes fusion of the exterior cell membrane with membranes of granules containing inflammatory mediators. Preformed granule contents, for example, histamine and heparin, dissolve and are released rapidly (within 5 minutes) while arachidonic acid metabolites, for example, leukotrienes and prostaglandins, are newly generated and released slightly later (5–30 minutes). These mediators increase vascular permeability and cause smooth muscle contraction.

Vaccines contain the active (label) antigens, often adjuvants, antibiotics, preservatives, residual culture medium proteins, and additives. Any vaccine component or excipient could potentially be responsible for an IgE-mediated reaction. In people, allergy to egg protein has been a major cause of allergic reaction after immunization,[18,19] and gelatin (likely of bovine or porcine origin) has also been incriminated as a cause of anaphylaxis.[20,21] Selected vaccines contain antibiotics, and drug sensitivities to neomycin, polymyxin B, amphotericin B, or penicillin have been responsible for vaccine-associated type I reactions. Latex from vaccine vial rubber stoppers and sorbitol can also evoke reactions. Adjuvants may have more of a secondary role by effecting T_H2 cells' response to the primary allergen.[22]

In a retrospective cohort study of more than a million dogs, risk factors were investigated for adverse events documented within 3 days of vaccination.[5] Most events were recorded the same day as the vaccination, with clinical signs consistent with type I hypersensitivity. Greatest risk was associated with the total number of vaccines, that is, milliliters of vaccine, received at the office visit, and a dose-response relationship was evident. The dose response was modified, however, by the dog's body weight, as the (%) increase in adverse event rate for each additional milliliter of vaccine in small (<10 kg) dogs was more than double the rise in rate seen in larger dogs. Even when number of vaccines and quantity were restricted, that is, dogs received only a 1-ml rabies vaccine, small dogs had a greater reaction rate than large dogs and a much greater rate than giant-breed dogs. Multivalent vaccines did not have a higher reaction rate than monovalent vaccines in this study.

Several different proteins have been purported as causes of vaccine-associated immediate hypersensitivity reactions in dogs and cats, even though most studies have not measured antigen-specific IgE concentrations. Without this important information, causes remain largely speculative. Most vaccines have been incriminated, but bacterial or spirochete vaccines may pose a higher risk. In Japan, Ohmori and colleagues[23] investigated IgE reactivity against fetal calf serum, gelatin, casein, and peptone in 10 dogs that exhibited allergic reactions at vaccination and compared the results to that of 50 vaccinated but asymptomatic dogs. Seven of 10 dogs with reactions had significantly increased IgE reactivity against fetal calf serum, a component of culture media used in vaccine production. Their analysis of vaccines found high concentrations of bovine serum albumin (BSA) in many vaccines.

A similar continuing study at Purdue University evaluated antigen-specific IgE response to BSA, casein, collagen I, bovine fibronectin, thyroglobulin, laminin, and porcine myosin in vaccinated dogs with or without an allergic reaction. IgE response against specific antigens was demonstrated in both the symptomatic and the asymptomatic group, with significant differences found only between matched samples, that is, littermates.[24] This IgE response in clinically normal dogs is consistent with laboratory studies in dogs[25] and indicates that an elevated antigen-specific IgE response by itself is not sufficient to cause clinical disease.

These study findings strongly suggest that vaccine excipients, probably common to many vaccines and manufacturing processes, are the most frequent allergens in canine and feline vaccines. For dogs, these proteins may be of bovine origin. It is not known whether protein exposure via diet (even exposure in utero or by nursing via the dam's diet) influences the development of specific IgE antibodies. This may, however, help explain allergic reactions occurring at the puppy's first vaccination.

Breed predispositions have been identified in large studies, with greatest risk noted for dachshunds, pugs, Boston terriers, miniature pinschers, and Chihuahuas. Among medium- to large-size breeds, boxers were at disproportionately greater risk.[5] Genetic differences exist, however, within breeds, and multiple genes or genetic regions are likely associated with manifestations of hypersensitivity. Identification of specific gene mutations may be too complex, in the near term, to be of practical significance. Nevertheless, the number of vaccines simultaneously administered to high-risk dogs should be minimized. Whether spacing vaccinations apart (and reducing incidence risk) reduces lifetime (cumulative) risk of a reaction is not known.

For humans, it is now advised that most patients with vaccine allergy can be safely vaccinated,[26] but the guidelines also recommend patient evaluation by an allergist or immunologist to define the suspected offending antigen. For animals with a history of anaphylaxis after vaccination, skin testing by intradermal inoculation of 0.1 ml of vaccine may elicit urticaria/wheal. Intradermal injections (0.1 ml) of a positive (histamine) and negative (saline) control are also needed for a comparison. If skin testing is not performed, high-risk patients can be premedicated with a H_1 antihistamine, for example, diphenhydramine, by subcutaneous or intramuscular administration at least 15 minutes before vaccination. For reasons unclear, not all patients with demonstrated hypersensitivity have reactions at their next vaccination (even without premedication), but owners should be counseled about risk and watchfulness for a reaction.

Clinical manifestations of immediate hypersensitivity in dogs are often related to the skin and general circulation, with signs of facial or periorbital edema, pruritus, wheals, hypotensive shock, or collapse. Vomiting, with or without diarrhea, and respiratory distress are less common in dogs. Cats often exhibit gastrointestinal and respiratory signs, including ptyalism, vomiting, and hemorrhagic diarrhea, as well as dyspnea, collapse, and facial swelling.

Treatment of type I reactions should be tailored to the type and severity of clinical signs. Indicated drugs (used alone or often in combination) include (1) H_1 antihistamines to block histamine receptors in immediate phase, (2) rapidly soluble glucocorticoids to block arachidonic pathways in late phase and shock, (3) epinephrine to relax smooth muscle, and (4) intravenous crystalloid fluids to combat hypotensive shock. Although not indicated for all patients, epinephrine and supplemental oxygen should be administered to patients with respiratory distress and cyanosis.

Type II

Type II hypersensitivity reactions are a consequence of IgG and IgM antibodies binding to specific cell surface antigens and producing cytotoxicity. These antibodies can interact with Fc receptors on effector cells such as neutrophils, NK cells, and mononuclear phagocytes, leading to target cell lysis by the effector cell. The attached antibody can also activate the complement pathway. While complement components C3a and C5a attract and activate other effector cells, components C3b, C3d, and the membrane attack complex (C5b-9) are deposited on target cell surfaces. Complement-mediated lysis may then occur, intravascularly destroying the target cell, or the cell may be removed extravascularly through opsonization and phagocytosis by splenic macrophages and Kupffer cells.

Immune-mediated cytotoxicity in companion animals is typically directed toward host platelets and/or erythrocytes, and dogs are much more commonly affected than cats. The diagnosis of immune-mediated cytotoxic disease is poorly defined in small animal practice, often becoming a diagnosis of exclusion. Available assays for antierythrocyte or antiplatelet antibodies have limited accuracy because of false-negative and false-positive results. A positive test is supportive of the diagnosis, but test sensitivity can be influenced by reagents and temperature.[27]

Immune-mediated thrombocytopenia, or idiopathic thrombocytopenic purpura (ITP), is an uncommon but known adverse vaccinal event following human immunization. The incidence is best recognized after measles-mumps-rubella immunization, although it has been reported after administration of other vaccines, such as hepatitis B, influenza, and varicella.[28,29] Postvaccinal ITP appears to be more likely after vaccination for viral diseases in which thrombocytopenia occurs during natural infection, for example, measles. Thrombocytopenia after routine immunization of children is usually benign, resolving within 1 month in most children.[30]

Immune-mediated hemolytic anemia (IMHA) or aplastic anemia from destruction of red cell precursors is considered an extremely rare sequela to human immunization.[29]

Although isolated cases have been reported,[31] it is unknown if the incidence is greater than the background rate for the disease.

Thrombocytopenia has been reported after modified live canine distemper virus vaccine administration in dogs, but the condition spontaneously resolved.[32] Whether the decreased platelet count was due to transient immune mechanisms or infectious mechanisms was unknown. Severe immune-mediated thrombocytopenia with petechiae has been stated to occur within 2 weeks of vaccination,[33] but cause or frequencies are unreported. It is unusual in practice to evaluate platelet counts within 2 weeks of vaccination, thus minor and transient decreases are rarely detected. More severe disease, necessitating glucocorticoid therapy, when seen in practice typically does not present with a history of recent vaccination. That would be expected because, under a uniform distribution, the 3 weeks following vaccination constitute only 5.8% (and 2 weeks only 3.8%) of an annual period. Better surveillance is needed to improve the understanding of the relationship of this disease to vaccination, but improved diagnostic tests are also required to identify an immune mechanism.

Vaccination has been a purported cause of IMHA in dogs, in spite of its rarity in cats and humans. This possible association was suggested by a case-control study in which 15 of 58 IMHA cases (26%) had been vaccinated in the previous 30 days compared with 5% of the 70 control dogs.[34] The second highest rate was among dogs (13 of 58) that were vaccinated more than 12 months before IMHA diagnosis. This association was not supported by a later case-control study which found no significant difference between groups.[35] Five (10%) of 52 cases had been vaccinated in the month before diagnosis, as had an equal number of control dogs. The largest number (17) of cases had been vaccinated 12 months or more before diagnosis, compared with 5 controls. Other investigators also failed to find an association between vaccination and IMHA using a case-control study.[36] Vaccination histories were not detailed in any of these studies.

Case-control studies are a reasonable and economical method to investigate rare events, but they need to be thorough. In different studies, and even within a study, dogs had been previously exposed to a myriad of vaccine antigens by way of different vaccinations from different manufacturers. Lack of detailed vaccination histories for the cases and controls reduces the ability to discern the predisposing factors (what loaded the gun?) as well as the precipitating, or antigen-specific, causes (what pulled the trigger?) of these adverse events. Due to the large number of marketed biologicals, large studies would likely be required to detect differences between groups. Vaccination may be an inciting cause of IMHA in some dogs, but probably not in most cases of IMHA. The extent to which that risk is increased with selected vaccine antigens is unknown.

The role of other autoantibodies and disease following vaccination is debated.[37] The mere detection or measurement of autoantibodies does not infer clinical disease. Does antibody production after vaccination account for canine immune-mediated thyroiditis and clinical hypothyroidism in dogs? A small experimental study showed that anticanine thyroglobulin antibodies were increased in dogs receiving a rabies vaccine, but not in dogs receiving only a multivalent distemper vaccine. When followed for almost 6 years, however, there was no difference in thyroid histopathology between vaccine groups and unvaccinated controls.[38,39]

Type III

Type III hypersensitivity reactions develop from acute inflammation triggered by the presence of immune complexes in tissues. Type III reactions differ from type II reactions in that type III reactions involve antibodies directed against soluble antigens in serum or tissues, producing antigen-antibody complexes. The antigen-antibody complexes subsequently invoke a variety of inflammatory processes as the antibodies engage Fc receptors on neutrophils, lymphocytes, basophils, and platelets. This process releases vasoactive amines, causing endothelial cell retraction, increasing vascular permeability, and allowing immune complex deposition on the vascular wall. Immune complexes also activate complement pathways, releasing peptides C3a and C5a and chemotactic factors. Macrophages are also stimulated by the complexes to release cytokines, such as TNF-α and IL-1, further inciting inflammation.

Clinical signs associated with type III reactions often become apparent with the rise of neutralizing antibody titers. Anterior uveitis, or blue eye, in dogs was associated with administration of modified live canine adenovirus type 1 (CAV-1) vaccines,[40] due to immune complex deposition in the anterior chamber and endothelial damage to the cornea. This problem has been virtually eliminated by the use of cross-protecting adenovirus type 2 (instead of CAV-1) in canine vaccines.

In many naturally occurring infectious diseases, immune complexes are deposited in the glomeruli. Glomerulonephritis has been noted in dogs and cats secondary to viral, rickettsial, and Dirofilarial infections. In spite of this, glomerulonephritis has not been attributed to complex deposition secondary to vaccination in dogs or cats. Renal disease is common in older cats, albeit usually interstitial, and recurrent vaccination has been postulated as a possible insidious cause. The use of feline kidney cell lines in production of vaccine for cats supports the biologic plausibility of vaccine-induced antibody formation against kidney cells, but experimental evidence is lacking. Although parental vaccination against feline viral rhinotracheitis, calicivirus, and panleukopenia can induce detectable antibodies against cell lysates, no renal disease was detected in a 56-week follow-up study.[41,42]

In people, immune complex deposition and associated joint disease can be a frequent but late complication of autoimmune disease, that is, rheumatoid arthritis. Although the role of vaccination in inciting or exacerbating this disease in humans has been debated,[43] it has not been proven. Due to the very low incidence of autoimmune disease in companion animals, a possible impact of vaccination on immune complex-related joint disease in dogs or cats remains unknown. A described immune-mediated polyarthritis in related young Akita dogs has several clinical signs similar to human juvenile rheumatoid arthritis, but lack of long-term follow-up in these dogs precluded determining any role of immune complex disease.[44] As noted with virtually any diagnosis in a young pet of vaccination age, a temporal association can be found but true pathophysiologic mechanisms secondary to vaccination remain unknown. This temporal relationship has been noted in a small case series of idiopathic immune-mediated polyarthritis,[45] but was not found in a larger group.[46]

Type IV

Type IV or delayed hypersensitivity, according to the Gell and Coombs classification, takes more than 12 hours to develop and involves a cell-mediated immune response rather than antibody response to antigens. Delayed hypersensitivity therefore indicates the presence of antigen-specific CD4 T cells. After activation, these T cells release proinflammatory cytokines, such as interferon-γ, TNF, IL-3, and granulocyte-macrophage colony-stimulating factor, which attract and activate macrophages. Chronic stimulation of T cells and cytokine release can result in the formation of granulomas, composed of macrophages and lymphocytes.

CUTANEOUS VASCULITIS OR GRANULOMATOUS REACTIONS

Dermatopathies have been reported to occur several weeks or months after vaccination. In 1986, pathologists reported a case series of 13 dogs with focal alopecia at sites of rabies vaccination.[47] Lesions were characterized by nonsuppurative inflammation and adnexal atrophy in the dermis and periarteriolar aggregates of lymphocytes and plasma cells in the subcutis. The arteritis was postulated to result from local formation of antigen-antibody complexes. Skin biopsies from 3 dogs were tested and had low-to-moderate intensity rabies-specific fluorescence in the walls of dermal blood vessels; skin biopsies from rabies-vaccinated asymptomatic dogs were not examined for comparison. Of the 13 affected dogs, 10 were poodles, and vaccines from at least 2 manufacturers were identified from case histories.

Subsequently, a pathology report of focal granulomatous panniculitis in 8 cats and 2 dogs documented deep dermal aggregates of macrophages, lymphocytes, plasma cells, and eosinophils at subcutaneous sites of rabies vaccination.[48] Four of the 10 cases also had discernible foreign material within macrophage cytoplasm, interpreted as vaccine-related material. More extensive immunologic tests were not performed.

Three mature dogs of different breeds with rabies vaccination-site alopecia later developed multifocal (pinnal margins, periocular areas, tail tip, and/or paw pads) cutaneous disease.[49] Ischemic dermatopathy was diagnosed based on reduced number and lymphocytic cuffing of dermal vessels, as well as a folliculocentric vasculopathy. Complement (C5b-9) deposition was observed in vessels of skeletal muscle in 2 of the dogs. The histologic changes in the dogs were noted to be indistinguishable from familial canine dermatomyositis. The specific antigenic stimulus for the complement-mediated microangiopathy was unknown, but microbial superantigens, as noted from disease after natural viral or bacterial infections, were postulated.

Clinical signs associated with ischemic vasculopathy were improved after oral pentoxifylline administration. Pentoxifylline is a methylxanthine derivative formulated for vasculopathic disease in people. It inhibits platelet and leukocyte adhesion to endothelial surfaces, improves erythrocyte flexibility, and reduces erythrocyte fragmentation, thus improving tissue perfusion. It may also have antiinflammatory effects by inhibiting TNF-α production.[50]

As noted with other adverse vaccinal events, specific vaccine components and mechanisms that serve as the predisposing or precipitating causes of this condition are unknown.

VACCINATION SITE–ASSOCIATED SARCOMAS

Fibrosarcomas and, to a much lesser degree, other soft tissue sarcomas have received much attention in feline practice and small animal vaccinology since the 1990s. Pathologists first reported an increase in the incidence of sarcomas diagnosed at vaccination sites in cats, with a speculated relationship to increased rabies vaccinations.[51,52] Contributing or associated factors at that time included an increasing cat population in the United States, advancements in feline practice, promotion of new feline vaccines, including feline leukemia virus (FeLV), and new local laws mandating vaccination of cats against rabies. Without a national database or mandatory reporting of adverse events, subsequent studies could only estimate prevalence. Estimates had wide (>10-fold) variation, ranging from as many as 1 in1000 vaccines administered to less than 1 in 10,000 vaccines.[53] Sarcomas in cats occur at rates much lower than immediate hypersensitivity, but are devastating in outcome because of their poor response to surgical or medical therapy.

Individual and collective efforts, including a national task force, sought to define the pathogenesis of this disease. Although initially associated with rabies vaccination sites, later studies found that FeLV vaccination posed equal or greater risk than rabies.[54,55] Sarcoma formation, however, has also been associated with other vaccines, and even with injection of nonbiologicals. A possible "smoking gun" emerged with the identification of aluminum in some of the described tumors.[52] Aluminum, as aluminum hydroxide or aluminum phosphate, is used as an adjuvant in some vaccines. Although there are other types of adjuvants, the particulate structure of aluminum makes it a readily identifiable marker of previous vaccination.

As discussed before, adjuvants enhance antigen presentation and potentiate the immune response. The degree and manner by which this response occurs varies with the structure and properties of the adjuvant and with the adsorption mechanism.[56,57] One theory is that overzealous inflammatory reactions to vaccine adjuvants promote vaccine-associated sarcomas. Adjuvanted vaccines produce histologically and sometimes grossly evident inflammation after vaccination,[58] but an association between overt localized reactions postvaccination and later sarcoma development had not been demonstrated.[16] Furthermore, no difference in sarcoma rates at sites of adjuvanted versus nonadjuvanted vaccine was reported in a large cohort of cats.[59]

Oncogenesis may be more related to inappropriate (and less overt) inflammatory reactions from which some fibroblasts undergo malignant transformation. Oncogenes may code for and overexpress growth factors or their receptors. Immunoreactivity for platelet-derived growth factor, epidermal growth factor, and their receptors and transforming growth factor β has been demonstrated in vaccine-associated sarcomas.[60] These investigators also found overexpression of c-jun, coding for translational protein AP-1 and implicated in stimulation of quiescent fibroblasts and oncogenesis.

The increased incidence of sarcomas may be due, largely or in part, to increased immunologic stimulation (via well-intended, repeated vaccination) of a genetically at-risk feline population. Immunohistochemical staining of feline vaccine-associated sarcomas revealed that most tumors had antibody staining for p53 mutation,[61] with nucleotide polymorphisms in the p53 gene sequence subsequently detected and associated with prognosis.[62] Tumor suppressor gene p53 encodes a nuclear protein involved in cell cycle regulation. Cells with mutated or absent p53 proceed unregulated through the cell cycle, creating aberrant clones and resulting in tumorigenesis. Specific p53 genotypes are likely associated with cancer phenotypes, and in humans, p53 mutation carriers have a greater than 100-fold risk of developing soft tissue sarcomas compared with noncarriers.[63]

Whereas much of the specific mechanisms related to immune response and genetic interaction remain to be determined, some veterinarians note that "the suggestive term 'vaccination-site fibrosarcoma' has been used a little too indiscriminately and has biased the veterinary and lay community alike."[64] This may lead to reduced vaccination against infectious diseases and subsequent loss of individual as well as herd immunity.

NEUROLOGIC COMPLICATIONS

Vaccine-induced neurologic disease is typically caused by the use of modified live virus vaccine and the recrudescence of a neurotropic agent, for example, rabies or canine distemper virus, producing clinical signs of that specific viral disease. The vaccine virus that is responsible for the disease can often be isolated from the sick patient. Multiple vaccines, or concurrent natural exposure to other pathogens, may exert an immunomodulating effect and increase susceptibility for this uncommon phenomenon.[65]

Immune-mediated neurologic disease is a rare adverse vaccinal event in human medicine. Guillain-Barré syndrome (GBS) is an autoimmune disease resulting from antibodies that cross-react with epitopes on peripheral nerves, for example, gangliosides, leading to nerve damage. GBS clinically presents as an acute flaccid paralysis, characterized by varying degrees of weakness, sensory abnormalities, and autonomic dysfunction.[66] About two-thirds of cases occur several days or weeks after a naturally occurring illness, often respiratory or enteric infections.[67] Vaccines have been temporally associated with the development of GBS in humans, with strongest evidence for swine flu (H1N1) vaccine in 1976–77 and older rabies vaccines.[37,68] This association has not been demonstrated with recent influenza vaccines.[69] Although polyradiculoneuropathies occur in companion animals and coonhound paralysis has been considered as an animal model of GBS,[70–72] reported associations between vaccination and this type of disease are quite rare in dogs or cats.[73,74] Specific immune mechanisms were not elucidated in these isolated case reports. In spite of a proposed autoimmune mechanism, glucocorticoids have not been shown effective in altering clinical signs of polyradiculoneuropathy; the immunosuppressive drug cyclophosphamide may alleviate disease severity.[33]

VACCINE-ASSOCIATED HYPERTROPHIC OSTEOPATHY (METAPHYSEAL OSTEODYSTROPHY)

Painful swelling of the distal radius/ulna (or less commonly, other long bones) with radiographic changes consistent with hypertrophic osteodystrophy (HOD) have been noted in young dogs within a week or two of vaccination. Because of the location of radiographic changes, this disease has also been termed metaphyseal osteopathy. Although also documented in small breeds, growing dogs of large or giant breeds seem more commonly affected. Great Danes, Irish setters, German shepherds, and Weimaraners are reported to have increased risk of HOD,[75] and the disease in Weimaraners has been more extensively investigated.[76–80] The described breed and familial tendencies support a genetic basis to the disease, but specific genes or genetic markers have not been identified.

Although recent vaccination is often reported in symptomatic puppies, the disease occurs in unvaccinated dogs.[79] With the disease most common in young dogs, it is not surprising that vaccinations were recently administered. Modified live canine distemper virus vaccines have also been associated with the disease,[33] but controlled studies have not evaluated relative risk compared with other vaccines. Without a control or comparison group, the exact role of vaccination will remain difficult to determine. Vaccination in a genetically susceptible dog possibly provides the immunologic stimulus to manifest clinical disease. Different vaccines (with their associated components) and the frequency/spacing of administration may modify the occurrence of disease.[77]

Clinical signs besides metaphyseal swelling and lameness can include fever and lymphadenopathy, with leukocytosis noted on complete blood count. Pyoderma and diarrhea are less commonly observed. Because postvaccinal concerns have been typically associated with the onset of juvenile bone disease and/or pyrexia, decreased neutrophil phagocytosis has not been suspected in these dogs, even though reported in young Weimaraners with recurrent infections.[81] Immunologic studies in Weimaraners found affected dogs to have lower concentrations of one or more serum immunoglobulins (IgG, IgM, and IgA); accurate vaccination histories were available on 10 dogs, and 9 had developed clinical signs within 5 days of a vacci-nation.[80] More extensive immunologic studies in postvaccinal affected dogs and in postvaccinal asymptomatic dogs (for comparison) are lacking. Investigators evalu-ating the findings, as well as response to therapy, have suggested that the clinical signs are manifestations of a form of immune dysregulation rather than a multifocal inflammatory disease.

Best recommendations for treatment are hindered by the lack of randomized clinical trials. Such trials should, in theory, be large enough to equally distribute between treat-ment groups patients that will likely vary in genetic predisposition, quality and quantity of immune stimulus, and degree and nature of immune dysregulation. This biologic variability somewhat explains differences in published treatment recommendations. Primary complaints of lameness with joint (or near-joint) swelling and radiographic changes in bone have supported guidance to administer NSAIDs,[82,83] which are effec-tive in some dogs. Concurrent fever and leukocytosis in affected dogs also raises concern of an infectious process and an understandable reluctance to use corticoste-roids. Nevertheless, glucocorticoids are the recommended treatment and are likely to give a superior response,[33,76,80] particularly when HOD presents soon after the immune stimulus of a vaccination. Antiinflammatory doses of glucocorticoids (0.5–1.0 mg/kg/d prednisolone) may be adequate for some cases, but high-dose pulse therapy (an immunosuppressive dose of 2–4 mg/kg/d tapered within a week to phys-iologic doses) can produce dramatic improvement in moderate and severe cases by rapidly downregulating steroid receptors and by inhibiting cytokine synthesis.

Are these dogs with suspected immune dysregulation at risk for other immune-related diseases after vaccination? Dogs with multiple manifestations of immunodefi-ciency, for example, stomatitis, and recurrent fever, will likely have disease problems regardless of vaccination. There is no long-term study of dogs with only HOD after vaccination. Recurrence of HOD appears to be unlikely after the dog's growth phase, and the (relative) immune stimulus from vaccination is likely reduced as a result of the increased body mass at adulthood. Nevertheless, restricting the number and type of vaccines administered to these dogs is prudent.[33]

SUMMARY

Adverse vaccinal events, or perceived vaccine-associated adverse events, are rela-tively uncommon after canine and feline vaccination. Nevertheless, undesired immune sequelae occur, often evoking great concern from owners and attending veterinarians. Because of the low incidence of these events and the large number of potential anti-genic causes, exact mechanisms may be difficult to elucidate. Good scientific studies, genetic studies to identify populations and breeds at risk, improved vaccine quality, and modified vaccination protocols will likely work together to further reduce these events in the future.

REFERENCES

1. Bradford-Hill AB. The environment and disease: association and causation. Proc R Soc Med 1965;58:295–300.
2. Siev D. An introduction to analytical methods for the postmarketing surveillance of veterinary vaccines. Adv Vet Med 1999;41:749–74.
3. Frana TS, Clough NE, Gatewood DM, et al. Postmarketing surveillance of rabies vaccines for dogs to evaluate safety and efficacy. J Am Vet Med Assoc 2008; 232(7):1000–2.

4. Moore GE, Frana TS, Guptill LF, et al. Postmarketing surveillance for dog and cat vaccines: new resources in changing times. J Am Vet Med Assoc 2005;227(7): 1066–9.

5. Moore GE, Guptill LF, Ward MP, et al. Adverse events diagnosed within three days of vaccine administration in dogs. J Am Vet Med Assoc 2005;227(7):1102–8.

6. Klein NP, Ray P, Carpenter D, et al. Rates of autoimmune diseases in Kaiser Permanente for use in vaccine adverse event safety studies. Vaccine 2009;28(4): 1062–8.

7. Reif DM, McKinney BA, Motsinger AA, et al. Genetic basis for adverse events after smallpox vaccination. J Infect Dis 2008;198(1):16–22.

8. Reif DM, Motsinger-Reif AA, McKinney BA, et al. Integrated analysis of genetic and proteomic data identifies biomarkers associated with adverse events following smallpox vaccination. Genes Immun 2009;10(2):112–9.

9. Castellino F, Galli G, Del Giudice G, et al. Generating memory with vaccination. Eur J Immunol 2009;39(8):2100–5.

10. Kang SM, Compans RW. Host responses from innate to adaptive immunity after vaccination: molecular and cellular events. Mol Cells 2009;27(1):5–14.

11. Medzhitov R, Janeway C Jr. Innate immune recognition: mechanisms and pathways. Immunol Rev 2000;173:89–97.

12. Akira S, Takeda K. Toll-like receptor signalling. Nat Rev Immunol 2004;4(7): 499–511.

13. Pashine A, Valiante NM, Ulmer JB. Targeting the innate immune response with improved vaccine adjuvants. Nat Med 2005;11(Suppl 4):S63–8.

14. Iwasaki A, Medzhitov R. Regulation of adaptive immunity by the innate immune system. Science 2010;327(5963):291–5.

15. Starr RM. Reaction rate in cats vaccinated with a new controlled-titer feline panleukopenia-rhinotracheitis-calicivirus-Chlamydia psittaci vaccine. Cornell Vet 1993;83(4):311–23.

16. Moore GE, DeSantis-Kerr AC, Guptill LF, et al. Adverse events after vaccine administration in cats: 2,560 cases (2002–2005). J Am Vet Med Assoc 2007; 231(1):94–100.

17. Ryan EP, Malboeuf CM, Bernard M, et al. Cyclooxygenase-2 inhibition attenuates antibody responses against human papillomavirus-like particles. J Immunol 2006;177(11):7811–9.

18. Georgitis JW, Fasano MB. Allergenic components of vaccines and avoidance of vaccination-related adverse events. Curr Allergy Rep 2001;1(1):11–7.

19. Nokleby H. Vaccination and anaphylaxis. Curr Allergy Asthma Rep 2006;6(1): 9–13.

20. Sakaguchi M, Inouye S. IgE sensitization to gelatin: the probable role of gelatin-containing diphtheria-tetanus-acellular pertussis (DTaP) vaccines. Vaccine 2000; 18(19):2055–8.

21. Pool V, Braun MM, Kelso JM, et al. Prevalence of anti-gelatin IgE antibodies in people with anaphylaxis after measles-mumps rubella vaccine in the United States. Pediatrics 2002;110(6):e71.

22. Trujillo-Vargas CM, Mayer KD, Bickert T, et al. Vaccinations with T-helper type 1 directing adjuvants have different suppressive effects on the development of allergen-induced T-helper type 2 responses. Clin Exp Allergy 2005;35(8): 1003–13.

23. Ohmori K, Masuda K, Maeda S, et al. IgE reactivity to vaccine components in dogs that developed immediate-type allergic reactions after vaccination. Vet Immunol Immunopathol 2005;104(3–4):249–56.

24. Moore GE, HogenEsch H, Dunham A. Antigenic causes of vaccine-associated allergic reactions in dogs. Proceedings of the 5th International Veterinary Vaccines and Diagnostics Conference. Madison (WI), July 19–23, 2009.
25. HogenEsch H, Dunham AD, Scott-Moncrieff C, et al. Effect of vaccination on serum concentrations of total and antigen-specific immunoglobulin E in dogs. Am J Vet Res 2002;63(4):611–6.
26. Kelso JM, Li JT, Nicklas RA, et al. Adverse reactions to vaccines. Ann Allergy Asthma Immunol 2009;103(4 Suppl 2):S1–14.
27. Warman SM, Murray JK, Ridyard A, et al. Pattern of Coombs' test reactivity has diagnostic significance in dogs with immune-mediated haemolytic anaemia. J Small Anim Pract 2008;49(10):525–30.
28. France EK, Glanz J, Xu S, et al. Risk of immune thrombocytopenic purpura after measles-mumps-rubella immunization in children. Pediatrics 2008;121(3):e687–92.
29. Schattner A. Consequence or coincidence? The occurrence, pathogenesis and significance of autoimmune manifestations after viral vaccines. Vaccine 2005; 23(30):3876–86.
30. Jadavji T, Scheifele D, Halperin S. Thrombocytopenia after immunization of Canadian children, 1992 to 2001. Pediatr Infect Dis J 2003;22(2):119–22.
31. Seltsam A, Shukry-Schulz S, Salama A. Vaccination-associated immune hemolytic anemia in two children. Transfusion 2000;40(8):907–9.
32. Straw B. Decrease in platelet count after vaccination with distemper-hepatitis (DH) vaccine. Vet Med Small Anim Clin 1978;73(6):725–6.
33. Greene CE, Schultz RD. Immunoprophylaxis. In: Greene CE, editor. Infectious diseases of the dog and cat. 3rd edition. Philadelphia: Elsevier Inc; 2006. p. 1069–119.
34. Duval D, Giger U. Vaccine-associated immune-mediated hemolytic anemia in the dog. J Vet Intern Med 1996;10(5):290–5.
35. Carr AP, Panciera DL, Kidd L. Prognostic factors for mortality and thromboembolism in canine immune-mediated hemolytic anemia: a retrospective study of 72 dogs. J Vet Intern Med 2002;16(5):504–9.
36. Klotins KC, Martin SW, Kruth S. Vaccination as a risk factor for immune mediated anemia in dogs: a multi-centre case-control study. Proceedings of the 3rd International Veterinary Vaccines and Diagnostics Conference. Guelph, Ontario (Canada), July 13–18, 2003.
37. Shoenfeld Y, Aron-Maor A. Vaccination and autoimmunity-'vaccinosis': a dangerous liaison? J Autoimmun 2000;14(1):1–10.
38. Scott-Moncrieff JC, Azcona-Olivera J, Glickman NW, et al. Evaluation of antithyroglobulin antibodies after routine vaccination in pet and research dogs. J Am Vet Med Assoc 2002;221(4):515–21.
39. Scott-Moncrieff JC, Glickman NW, Glickman LT, et al. Lack of association between repeated vaccination and thyroiditis in laboratory Beagles. J Vet Intern Med 2006;20(4):818–21.
40. Curtis R, Barnett KC. The 'blue eye' phenomenon. Vet Rec 1983;112(15):347–53.
41. Lappin MR, Basaraba RJ, Jensen WA. Interstitial nephritis in cats inoculated with Crandell Rees feline kidney cell lysates. J Feline Med Surg 2006;8(5):353–6.
42. Lappin MR, Jensen WA, Jensen TD, et al. Investigation of the induction of antibodies against Crandell-Rees feline kidney cell lysates and feline renal cell lysates after parenteral administration of vaccines against feline viral rhinotracheitis, calicivirus, and panleukopenia in cats. Am J Vet Res 2005;66(3):506–11.
43. Cohen AD, Shoenfeld Y. Vaccine-induced autoimmunity. J Autoimmun 1996;9(6): 699–703.

44. Dougherty SA, Center SA, Shaw EE, et al. Juvenile-onset polyarthritis syndrome in Akitas. J Am Vet Med Assoc 1991;198(5):849–56.
45. Kohn B, Garner M, Lubke S, et al. Polyarthritis following vaccination in four dogs. Vet Comp Orthop Traumatol 2003;16(1):6–10.
46. Clements DN, Gear RN, Tattersall J, et al. Type I immune-mediated polyarthritis in dogs: 39 cases (1997–2002). J Am Vet Med Assoc 2004;224(8):1323–7.
47. Wilcock BP, Yager JA. Focal cutaneous vasculitis and alopecia at sites of rabies vaccination in dogs. J Am Vet Med Assoc 1986;188(10):1174–7.
48. Hendrick MJ, Dunagan CA. Focal necrotizing granulomatous panniculitis associated with subcutaneous injection of rabies vaccine in cats and dogs: 10 cases (1988–1989). J Am Vet Med Assoc 1991;198(2):304–5.
49. Vitale CB, Gross TL, Magro CM. Vaccine-induced ischemic dermatopathy in the dog. Vet Dermatol 1999;10(2):131–42.
50. Alkharfy KM, Kellum JA, Matzke GR. Unintended immunomodulation: part II. Effects of pharmacological agents on cytokine activity. Shock 2000;13(5):346–60.
51. Hendrick MJ, Goldschmidt MH. Do injection site reactions induce fibrosarcomas in cats? J Am Vet Med Assoc 1991;199(8):968.
52. Hendrick MJ, Goldschmidt MH, Shofer FS, et al. Postvaccinal sarcomas in the cat: epidemiology and electron probe microanalytical identification of aluminum. Cancer Res 1992;52(19):5391–4.
53. McEntee MC, Page RL. Feline vaccine-associated sarcomas. J Vet Intern Med 2001;15(3):176–82.
54. Kass PH, Barnes WG Jr, Spangler WL, et al. Epidemiologic evidence for a causal relation between vaccination and fibrosarcoma tumorigenesis in cats. J Am Vet Med Assoc 1993;203(3):396–405.
55. Hendrick MJ, Shofer FS, Goldschmidt MH, et al. Comparison of fibrosarcomas that developed at vaccination sites and at nonvaccination sites in cats: 239 cases (1991–1992). J Am Vet Med Assoc 1994;205(10):1425–9.
56. Spickler AR, Roth JA. Adjuvants in veterinary vaccines: modes of action and adverse effects. J Vet Intern Med 2003;17(3):273–81.
57. Hem SL, Hogenesch H. Relationship between physical and chemical properties of aluminum-containing adjuvants and immunopotentiation. Expert Rev Vaccines 2007;6(5):685–98.
58. Day MJ, Schoon HA, Magnol JP, et al. A kinetic study of histopathological changes in the subcutis of cats injected with non-adjuvanted and adjuvanted multi-component vaccines. Vaccine 2007;25(20):4073–84.
59. Norsworthy GD. Counteracting the decline in feline visits and vaccinations. J Am Vet Med Assoc 2008;233(9):1397.
60. Hendrick MJ. Feline vaccine-associated sarcomas. Cancer Invest 1999;17(4):273–7.
61. Hershey AE, Dubielzig RR, Padilla ML, et al. Aberrant p53 expression in feline vaccine-associated sarcomas and correlation with prognosis. Vet Pathol 2005;42(6):805–11.
62. Banerji N, Kanjilal S. Somatic alterations of the p53 tumor suppressor gene in vaccine-associated feline sarcoma. Am J Vet Res 2006;67(10):1766–72.
63. Hwang SJ, Lozano G, Amos CI, et al. Germline p53 mutations in a cohort with childhood sarcoma: sex differences in cancer risk. Am J Hum Genet 2003;72(4):975–83.
64. Horzinek MC, Thiry E. Vaccines and vaccination: the principles and the polemics. J Feline Med Surg 2009;11(7):530–7.

65. Krakowka S, Olsen RG, Axthelm MK, et al. Canine parvovirus infection potentiates canine distemper encephalitis attributable to modified live-virus vaccine. J Am Vet Med Assoc 1982;180(2):137–9.

66. Vucic S, Kiernan MC, Cornblath DR. Guillain-Barre syndrome: an update. J Clin Neurosci 2009;16(6):733–41.

67. Hughes RA, Rees JH. Clinical and epidemiologic features of Guillain-Barre syndrome. J Infect Dis 1997;176(Suppl 2):S92–8.

68. Haber P, Sejvar J, Mikaeloff Y, et al. Vaccines and Guillain-Barre syndrome. Drug Saf 2009;32(4):309–23.

69. Greene SK, Kulldorff M, Lewis EM, et al. Near real-time surveillance for influenza vaccine safety: proof-of-concept in the vaccine safety datalink project. Am J Epidemiol 2010;171(2):177–88.

70. Cuddon PA. Electrophysiologic assessment of acute polyradiculoneuropathy in dogs: comparison with Guillain-Barre syndrome in people. J Vet Intern Med 1998;12(4):294–303.

71. Holmes DF, Schultz RD, Cummings JF, et al. Experimental coonhound paralysis: animal model of Guillain-Barre syndrome. Neurology 1979;29(8):1186–7.

72. Northington JW, Brown MJ. Acute canine idiopathic polyneuropathy. A Guillain-Barre-like syndrome in dogs. J Neurol Sci 1982;56(2–3):259–73.

73. Gehring R, Eggars B. Suspected post-vaccinal acute polyradiculoneuritis in a puppy. J S Afr Vet Assoc 2001;72(2):96.

74. Schrauwen E, van Ham L. Postvaccinal acute polyradiculoneuritis in a young puppy. Prog Vet Neurol 1995;6:68–70.

75. LaFond E, Breur GJ, Austin CC. Breed susceptibility for developmental orthopedic diseases in dogs. J Am Anim Hosp Assoc 2002;38(5):467–77.

76. Abeles V, Harrus S, Angles JM, et al. Hypertrophic osteodystrophy in six weimaraner puppies associated with systemic signs. Vet Rec 1999;145(5):130–4.

77. Harrus S, Waner T, Aizenberg I, et al. Development of hypertrophic osteodystrophy and antibody response in a litter of vaccinated Weimaraner puppies. J Small Anim Pract 2002;43(1):27–31.

78. Woodard JC. Canine hypertrophic osteodystrophy, a study of the spontaneous disease in littermates. Vet Pathol 1982;19(4):337–54.

79. Grondalen J. Metaphyseal osteopathy (hypertrophic osteodystrophy) in growing dogs. A clinical study. J Small Anim Pract 1976;17(11):721–35.

80. Foale RD, Herrtage ME, Day MJ. Retrospective study of 25 young weimaraners with low serum immunoglobulin concentrations and inflammatory disease. Vet Rec 2003;153(18):553–8.

81. Couto CG, Krakowka S, Johnson G, et al. In vitro immunologic features of Weimaraner dogs with neutrophil abnormalities and recurrent infections. Vet Immunol Immunopathol 1989;23(1–2):103–12.

82. Muir P, Dubielzig RR, Johnson KA, et al. Hypertrophic osteodystrophy and calvarial hyperostosis. Compend Contin Educ Pract Vet 1996;18(2):143–50.

83. Gilad J, Barnea E, Klement E. Aspirin treatment of postvaccinal hypertrophic osteodystrophy in a weimaraner puppy. Vet Rec 2002;150(14):456.

Immunodeficiencies Caused by Infectious Diseases

Jane E. Sykes, BVSc(Hons), PhD

KEYWORDS

- Feline immunodeficiency virus • Feline leukemia virus
- *Anaplasma phagocytophilum* • *Ehrlichia canis*
- Distemper virus • Parvovirus

The classic example of immunodeficiency caused by an infectious agent is the acquired immunodeficiency syndrome, caused by human immunodeficiency virus (HIV). Similarly, the best known pathogens of companion animals causing immunodeficiencies are the feline retroviruses feline immunodeficiency virus (FIV) and feline leukemia virus (FeLV). However, several other pathogens are capable of disrupting normal immune function. Many infectious agents disrupt host barriers to infection. This may result from the inflammatory response to a pathogen or direct damage by the microbe itself. Examples include disruption of the gastrointestinal mucosal barrier by canine parvovirus, destruction of nasal turbinates by *Aspergillus fumigatus* in canine sinonasal aspergillosis, or paralysis of the respiratory cilia by *Bordetella bronchiseptica*. *Anaplasma phagocytophilum* disables neutrophil function, ensuring its survival within a cell normally charged with antimicrobial substances. Viruses, such as canine distemper virus, cause lymphopenia; the outcome of infection depends on the balance between viral destruction of the immune system and the ability of the remaining immune defenses to eliminate the virus.

Disruption of immune function by infectious agents may serve to promote the infectious agent's survival through host immune evasion. Immunosuppression having the greatest impact clinically often occurs as a result of infection with organisms that are able to persist within the host. Ideally, a pathogen is able to adapt such that it can coexist with the host, without causing death of the host or severe illness, in a way that maximizes the pathogen's transmission efficiency.

The types of opportunistic infections that occur in patients that are immune compromised as a result of an underlying immunosuppressive infection depend upon the mechanisms of immunosuppression. Impairment of normal host barrier function or the function of granulocytes is generally associated with a broad spectrum of bacterial

Department of Medicine & Epidemiology, University of California, Davis, 2108 Tupper Hall, Davis, CA 95616, USA
E-mail address: jesykes@ucdavis.edu

Vet Clin Small Anim 40 (2010) 409–423
doi:10.1016/j.cvsm.2010.01.006
0195-5616/10/$ – see front matter. Published by Elsevier Inc.

infections and sometimes infection with opportunistic fungi, such as *Aspergillus* spp Impairment of cell-mediated immunity (CMI) results in infections with opportunistic pathogens, such as *Nocardia* spp, *Mycobacterium* spp, *Toxoplasma gondii*, and a variety of fungal pathogens. Reactivation of dormant pathogens, such as feline herpesvirus, may also occur with depression of CMI.

The purpose of this article is to highlight some of the mechanisms by which persistent infectious microorganisms cause acquired immunodeficiency in companion animal species, and the consequences of the resulting disturbance in immune function.

VIRAL INFECTIONS CAUSING IMMUNODEFICIENCY
Canine Distemper Virus Infection

Canine distemper virus (CDV) causes canine distemper, a common disease of dogs worldwide that is associated with a high degree of morbidity and mortality. The virus also infects several other species, including foxes, raccoons, skunks, ferrets, and free-ranging and captive felids. Disease in dogs is most prevalent in regions where vaccination of young dogs against the disease is either not performed or is poorly timed, and epidemics continue to occur in shelter environments in developed countries.[1]

Canine distemper virus is a Morbillivirus related to measles virus and has been used to study the pathogenesis of measles virus infection. Morbilliviruses are enveloped RNA viruses that survive poorly in the environment. Based on genetic variation within the viral hemagglutinin (H) gene, a multitude of different strains of CDV exist that vary in their geographic distribution, cell tropism, and virulence. Although CDV infects a variety of different cell types, including epithelial, mesenchymal, neuroendocrine, and hematopoietic cells, the marked tropism of CDV for immune cells is critical in respect to its ability to cause immunosuppression. Viral components involved in CDV-induced immunodeficiency include the viral hemagglutinin; the V protein (a nonstructural phosphoprotein); and the nucleocapsid (N) protein.

Dogs are generally exposed to CDV through contact with infected oronasal secretions. The virus initially infects monocytes within lymphoid tissue in the upper respiratory tract and tonsils and is subsequently disseminated via the lymphatics and blood to the entire reticuloendothelial system. Direct viral destruction of a significant proportion of the lymphocyte population, and especially CD4+ T cells, occurs within the blood, tonsils, thymus, spleen, lymph nodes, bone marrow, mucosa-associated lymphoid tissue, and the hepatic Kupffer cells.[1–3] This viral destruction is associated with an initial lymphopenia and transient fever that occurs a few days after infection. Subsequently, there is a second stage of cell-associated viremia, after which CDV infects cells of the lower respiratory; gastrointestinal tract; central nervous system; urinary tract; and red and white blood cells, including additional lymphoid cells.

Elimination of CDV by the host depends on humoral and CMI.[1,4] Because the virus is lymphocytolytic, the outcome of infection depends on the rate at which the host is able to remove the virus before the virus has sufficient time to cause severe immune system injury. Dogs mounting a partial immune response may undergo recovery from acute illness but fail to eliminate the virus completely, leading to a spectrum of more chronic disease manifestations that often involve the uvea, lymphoid organs, footpads, and especially the CNS. Opportunistic infections may also have the chance to develop in these dogs.

Dogs with canine distemper may develop profound lymphopenia and leucopenia. Lymphopenia results from generalized depletion of T and B cells in a variety of tissues

(**Fig. 1**). CD4+ T cells are preferentially depleted during the acute phase, which is followed by CD8+ cell depletion.[5,6] Necrosis of hematopoietic cells within the bone marrow may result in leucopenia.[7]

Infection of ferrets has been used as a model of CDV-induced immunosuppression.[8] CDV infection of ferrets leads to dramatic reduction in cell-mediated immune function with markedly depressed lymphocyte proliferative activity, and to some extent delayed type hypersensitivity responses. The virus enters lymphocytes following binding of the viral H gene to the primary receptor for the virus, signaling lymphocyte activation molecule (CD150, SLAM). The expression of SLAM appears to be upregulated in response to CDV infection.[9] SLAM is also expressed on antigen-presenting cells, such as dendritic cells and activated monocytes, and infection of these cells, which may predominate in the chronic phase of infection, has been hypothesized to be associated with impaired antigen presentation.[1,6] Infection of dendritic cells within the thymus may lead to impaired maturation and selection of T cells, with subsequent release of immature CD5- T cells, including cells that may have the potential for autoreactivity.[6] Lymphocyte apoptosis also occurs independent of viral infection in canine distemper, although the mechanisms have not yet been elucidated.[10] The presence of the viral V protein is essential to permit rapid replication of CDV in T cells and critical in CDV-mediated immunosuppression. This protein almost completely antagonizes alpha interferon, TNF-alpha, Il-6, gamma-interferon, and Il-2 in the acute phase of infection.[3] Suppression of the cytokine response is associated with severe immunosuppression and a fatal outcome in ferrets. Finally, the N protein of Morbilliviruses may interfere with the immune response through the binding of the CD32 (Fc-gamma) receptor on B cells, resulting in impaired differentiation of B cells into plasma cells.[11] Binding of this receptor on dendritic cells[12] is associated with impairment of antigen presentation by dendritic cells and resulting disruption of T cell function.

The most common secondary infections in canine distemper are secondary bacterial infections that contribute to bronchopneumonia. *Bordetella bronchiseptica* is also a common co-pathogen in dogs with distemper. Dogs may be diagnosed with bordetellosis in the early stages of distemper, the underlying CDV infection being overlooked. Other opportunistic infections that have been identified in dogs with distemper include toxoplasmosis,[13] salmonellosis,[14] nocardiosis,[15,16] and generalized demodicosis (Sykes and colleagues, unpublished observations, 2006). In one study from Brazil, canine distemper was the most common underlying immunosuppressive

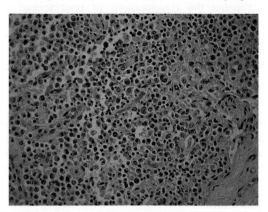

Fig. 1. Severe cortical lymphoid necrosis in a mandibular lymph node from a 5-month-old female spayed German Shepherd cross that was euthanized as a result of canine distemper virus infection.

disease predisposing to nocardiosis in dogs.[16] Infection with *Pneumocystis carinii* was associated with CDV infection in a mink,[17] and concurrent neosporosis and canine distemper was reported in a raccoon.[18]

Canine Parvovirus 2 and Feline Panleukopenia Virus Infection

Although parvoviruses do not cause chronic, persistent infections in dogs and cats, parvoviral replication creates the perfect storm for development of acute and severe opportunistic bacterial infections. The combination of leukopenia, disruption of the gastrointestinal barrier, and the immature immune system of the young animals that are most susceptible to these viruses is associated with the common development of sepsis, which is frequently the cause of death.

Canine parvovirus 2 (CPV-2) and feline panleukopenia virus (FPV) are small, nonenveloped DNA viruses. Since its emergence in 1978, CPV has subsequently mutated to CPV-2a; CPV-2b; and in the last decade, CPV-2c, which was first documented in Italy and has subsequently spread to dogs on every continent, with the exception of Australia. The CPV-2c strain appears to be particularly virulent and there has been some debate regarding the ability of current vaccines to protect against it and the ability of commercially available SNAP ELISA tests to detect the virus.[19]

CPV and FPV have tropism for rapidly dividing cells. As such, they exert an effect on the host that resembles the outcome of treatment with a chemotherapeutic drug. The virus binds and enters cells using the transferrin receptor.[20] Cells preferentially involved are the crypt cells of the gastrointestinal tract, bone marrow, and lymphoid tissue. Leukopenia results from sequestration of neutrophils within damaged gastrointestinal tissue and is compounded by destruction of white cell precursors within the bone marrow. Damage to the gastrointestinal barrier can result in translocation of enteric bacteria. In the face of the massive immunosuppression that ensues as a result of virus-induced neutropenia and lymphopenia, the host fails to contain bacterial replication and bacteremia and sepsis ensue. Treatment of secondary infections with broad-spectrum parenteral antimicrobial drugs is critical to permit recovery of dogs and cats from parvoviral infection. Bacterial causes of sepsis reported in infected animals include *Escherichia coli*, *Salmonella* spp, and *Clostridium difficile*. *Giardia* infection also exacerbates illness.[21] Immunosuppression may also contribute to replication of other co-infecting enteric viruses, such as enteric coronavirus, which in turn exacerbate the damage to the gastrointestinal mucosa. Similarly, CPV-induced immunosuppression potentiates the development of postvaccinal canine distemper encephalitis.[22]

The importance of secondary infections in the pathogenesis of parvovirus infections is highlighted by the fact that experimental infection of germfree cats is not associated with development of clinical illness, despite the associated reduction in white cell count.[23]

Feline Retroviral Infections

Feline leukemia virus and feline immunodeficiency virus are common causes of viral-induced immunodeficiency in cats, although the underlying mechanisms by which they exert immunodeficiency are still incompletely understood. Subtypes of FeLV and FIV are defined based on variations in the *env* gene sequence, which also influences their pathogenicity.

Feline Leukemia Virus Infection

There are four different subtypes of the gamma retrovirus FeLV: FeLV-A, FeLV-B, FeLV-C, and FeLV-T. Each subtype uses a different receptor to enter cells (**Table 1**).[24–27] All cats infected with FeLV-B, FeLV-C, and FeLV-T are co-infected with FeLV-A, with FeLV-A being the only type that is transmitted between animals. The other subtypes arise through recombination or point mutation within FeLV-A during the course of infection and influence the clinical expression of disease (see **Table 1**). FeLV-T, a T-cell tropic variant, is unique amongst gamma retroviruses in that it requires two host proteins to enter and infect cells.[27] As a result of its T-cell tropism, FeLV-T infection may be particularly associated with immunodeficiency in cats.

Transmission of FeLV-A primarily occurs through prolonged, close contact with salivary secretions, although other routes of transmission, including through biting, can also occur. After an initial phase of viremia, FeLV replicates within rapidly dividing lymphoid, myeloid, and epithelial cells, such as those lining the intestinal crypts.[28] As with distemper, when cellular destruction exceeds the ability of the host's immune system to suppress viral replication, persistent viremia and progressive FeLV-related disease results.

Clinical outcomes of FeLV infection include tumor development, especially lymphoma or leukemia; non-regenerative anemia; marrow failure, which in turn can result from myelophthisis, myelodysplasia, or myelofibrosis; neurologic manifestations, such as anisocoria; reproductive failure; gastrointestinal disease; and immunodeficiency. The development of opportunistic infections may result from marrow failure or cell-mediated immunodeficiency. The immunosuppressive properties of FeLV have been linked at least in part to the transmembrane viral envelope peptide,

Table 1
Host cellular receptors involved in FeLV infection

FeLV Subtype	Receptor	Receptor Function	Comments	References
FeLV-A	FeTHTR1	Thiamine transporter protein	Present in all cats with FeLV; transmitted exogenously	Mendoza et al[24]
FeLV-B	FePit1 or FePit2	Inorganic phosphate transporter protein	Results from recombination between FeLV-A and feline endogenous FeLV-related retrovirus sequences; may accelerate development of lymphoma or enhance neuropathogenicity	Anderson et al[25]
FeLV-C	FLVCR	Heme transporter protein	Arises from point mutations in FeLV-A *env* gene; associated with non-regenerative anemia	Keel et al[26]
FeLV-T	FePit1 or FLVCR *plus* a soluble cofactor encoded by endogenous FeLV-related retrovirus sequence, usually FeLIX	Transporter protein (variable)	Arises from point mutations in FeLV-A *env* gene; associated with severe immunosuppression	Anderson[27]

p15E.[29] This viral protein inhibits T- and B-cell function, inhibits cytotoxic lymphocyte responses, alters monocyte morphology and distribution, and has been associated with impaired cytokine production and responsiveness.[30–32] Kittens persistently infected with FeLV have impaired T-cell, and to a lesser extent, B-cell function.[33–36] Infected cats may develop lymphopenia, thymic atrophy, and depletion of lymphocytes within lymph node paracortical zones. CD4+ T-cell malfunction may contribute to a decreased humoral and cellular immune response in affected cats.[37,38] The response to vaccination may also be impaired. Neutrophil function is also impaired in cats that are FeLV-infected.[39–41] Opportunistic infections documented in cats that are FeLV-infected include bacterial infections of the upper and lower urinary tract, hemoplasmosis, respiratory tract infections, feline infectious peritonitis (FIP), and chronic stomatitis, although there is little evidence in the literature to support an increased prevalence of these infections in cats with FeLV as opposed to cats not infected with FeLV. Some infections, such as cryptococcosis, appear to occur with the same frequency in cats that are FeLV positive as in cats that are FeLV negative, but may be more severe and refractory to therapy (**Fig. 2**).[42]

Feline Immunodeficiency Virus Infection

FIV is a lentivirus that is primarily transmitted between cats by biting. FIV invades cells via the primary receptor CD134, which is expressed on feline CD4+ T lymphocytes; B lymphocytes; activated macrophages[43,44]; and the secondary receptor CXCR4, a chemokine receptor.

The mechanisms of immunosuppression in FIV infection are complex, and despite more than 20 years of research on the subject, not completely understood. Paradoxically, immune suppression and immune hyperactivation have been documented in infected cats. A comprehensive review of the subject is beyond the scope of this article but has been recently published elsewhere.[45]

Central to FIV-induced immunosuppression is a progressive reduction in CD4+ T-cell numbers. The number of CD4+ T cells in peripheral blood declines shortly after infection, owing to initial viral replication within target activated CD4+ T cells and macrophages. After this acute phase of infection, numbers of CD4+ T cells rebound and viremia is suppressed (**Fig. 3**). Neutropenia can also occur during this phase[46] and it has been suggested that this may result from neutrophil apoptosis.[47] CD4+/CD25+ T regulator cells have recently been shown to be infected and activated during acute

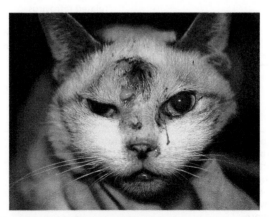

Fig. 2. Siamese cat with FeLV infection and concurrent severe cryptococcal rhinosinusitis that was refractory to therapy with antifungal drugs.

infection. When activated, these cells inhibit proliferation and induce apoptosis of other activated CD4+ or CD8+ T cells, which may also contribute to persistence of FIV and further immunosuppression.[45,48,49] Evidence also points to altered dendritic cell function during acute FIV infection.[50,51] The impairment of T-cell function in acute FIV infection has been suggested to result from cytokine dysregulation, immunologic anergy, and increased apoptosis.[45] In turn, this is associated with an inability to mount a primary immune response to opportunistic pathogens.

A prolonged asymptomatic period follows, sometimes lasting years or even the life-time of the cat, which is associated with a gradual decline in CD4+ T-cell numbers; a reduction in the CD4+/CD8+ ratio; generalized lymphoid depletion; and in some cats, hyperglobulinemia, which results from B-cell hyperactivation. In addition to a decline in cell numbers, although activated, paradoxically, T cells develop a reduced ability to respond to antigenic stimulation. Altered lymphocyte expression of cell surface molecules, including CD4, cytokine receptors and major histocompatibility complex (MHC) II antigens, and continued alteration of dendritic cell function, also contribute to immunosuppression. Dysregulation of cytokine production occurs. Cats chronically infected with FIV fail to produce Il-2, Il-6, and Il-12 in response to *T gondii* infection, instead producing elevated levels of the antiinflammatory cytokine Il-10.[45,52]

Ultimately these changes lead to opportunistic infections, most commonly bacterial infections of the mouth; chronic bacterial skin infections; persistent viral upper respiratory tract infections; mycobacterial infections; hemoplasmosis; toxoplasmosis; and parasitic infections, such as demodicosis and severe flea burdens.

Feline Coronavirus Infection

FIP virus infection is associated with a profound, virus-induced depletion of CD4+ and CD8+ cells and hypergammaglobulinemia, suggesting virus-induced dysregulation of

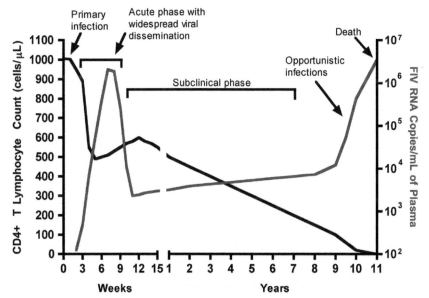

Fig. 3. Graph depicting the pathogenesis of feline immunodeficiency virus infection. As the CD4+ count declines, production of antibody is limited and cats with advanced infection may test negative using antibody tests. Opportunistic infections ensue.

the immune response.[53] The mechanism of T cell depletion is not clear, because the virus does not infect lymphocytes, only monocytes and macrophages. Infection of antigen-presenting cells, specifically dendritic cells, by the virus has been hypothesized to cause T-cell apoptosis.[53] Despite the profound T-cell deficiency that accompanies FIP, opportunistic infections are rarely reported, perhaps partly as a result of the rapidly fatal clinical course of disease.

BACTERIAL INFECTIONS CAUSING IMMUNODEFICIENCY

Perhaps the best examples of bacterial infections causing immunodeficiency are those of the tick-borne pathogens *Ehrlichia canis* and *Anaplasma phagocytophilum*, which are described later in this article. *Bartonella* spp. and hemotropic mycoplasmas (hemoplasmas) may also be capable of inducing chronic immunodeficiencies. Human infection with *Bartonella bacilliformis* infection may be immunosuppressive and many patients have succumbed with secondary bacterial infections, especially salmonellosis.[54] Impaired leukocyte function, cyclic CD8+ lymphopenia, and diminished expression of adhesion molecules and MHC Class II molecules by CD8+ and B lymphocytes, respectively, were documented in one study of *Bartonella vinsonii* subspecies *berkhoffii*-infected dogs.[55] Hemoplasma-induced immunosuppression is not a new phenomenon and has been recognized as a problem in experiments involving chronically infected laboratory rodents and in sheep chronically infected with *Mycoplasma ovis*.[56,57] The clinical importance of immunosuppression induced by *Bartonella* spp and hemoplasmas in cats and dogs requires further investigation.

Ehrlichia canis Infection

Ehrlichia canis is a gram negative intracellular bacteria that causes canine monocytic ehrlichiosis (CME), arguably the most important infectious disease of dogs exposed to ticks worldwide. The organism is transmitted by the brown dog tick, *Rhipicephalus sanguineus*. The organism infects monocytes, in which it forms morulae. In the United States, disease is diagnosed most frequently in dogs living in the southeastern and southwestern states, but because of chronic, subclinical infection, dogs can be transported to non-endemic regions and subsequently develop disease. Different strains of *E canis* exist but the degree by which these vary in virulence is poorly characterized.

The course of CME has been divided into acute, subclinical, and chronic phases, although in naturally infected dogs, these phases are often not readily distinguishable. Clinical signs of acute disease include depression, inappetence, fever, and weight loss. Ocular and nasal discharges, edema, hemorrhages, and neurologic signs may also occur. The organism replicates in reticuloendothelial cells with generalized lymphadenopathy and splenomegaly, and transient cytopenias, especially thrombocytopenia, may occur. After the acute phase, which may last up to 6 weeks, a subclinical phase may develop that lasts months to years. During this phase, the organism appears to evade host immune responses through antigenic variation. Ultimately, a small percentage of these infected dogs develop chronic CME. Chronic CME is characterized by signs that include lethargy, inappetence, fever, weight loss, bleeding tendencies, pallor, lymphadenopathy, splenomegaly, dyspnea, anterior uveitis, polyuria/polydipsia, muscle wasting, polyarthritis, and edema. Dogs with severe chronic ehrlichiosis may develop marrow failure, with aplastic pancytopenia. Severe disease may also be associated with a protein-losing nephropathy and development of neurologic signs. Some dogs have bone marrow plasmacytosis and peripheral granular lymphocytosis. Hyperglobulinemia is a frequent finding on the serum chemistry profile and usually results from a polyclonal gammopathy, although monoclonal gammopathies have also been reported.[58] High antibody titers to *E canis*, occasionally exceeding 1:1,000,000, are also common.

The chronic phase may also be associated with development of secondary opportunistic infections. The precise underlying mechanism of the immunodeficiency that develops and how it relates to successful persistence of *E canis* has not been elucidated. Not all dogs that develop chronic infections are pancytopenic, so leukopenia alone does not explain the predisposition for opportunistic infection. Furthermore, the types of infections reported, such as viral papillomatosis; generalized demodicosis; protozoal infections, such as neosporosis and opportunistic mycoses, suggest a defect develops in CMI (**Fig. 4**).[59] *E canis* infection has also been suggested to predispose dogs to development of canine leishmaniasis.[60] Infection of a canine cell line with *E canis* resulted in suppression of MHC Class II expression.[61] In one study, acute experimental infection with *E canis* was not associated with measurable suppression of CMI or humoral immune responses.[62] Alterations in immune responses during chronic infection require further evaluation.

Anaplasma Phagocytophilum Infection

Like *E canis*, *Anaplasma phagocytophilum* is an obligate, tick-transmitted intracellular bacteria that forms morulae within leukocytes. In contrast to *E canis* which infects monocytes, *A phagocytophilum* infects granulocytes, primarily the neutrophil,[63] and causes granulocytic anaplasmosis, a disease of humans, dogs, horses, ruminants, and occasionally cats (**Fig. 5**). The vector ticks are generally those belonging to the *Ixodes persulcatus* complex, primarily *I scapularis* and *I pacificus* in the United States, and *I ricinus* in Europe. Numerous small wild mammals, deer, and possibly birds, act as reservoir hosts for the organism. Several genetic variants have been identified and there is increasing evidence of strain variation in host specificity and pathogenicity.

Immunosuppression resulting from *A phagocytophilum* infection results primarily from impairment of neutrophil function by the bacteria. After inoculation into the host, *A phagocytophilum* attaches to sialylated ligands on the surface of neutrophils, after which it enters neutrophils via caveolae-mediated endocytosis, bypassing phagolysosomal pathways. *A phagocytophilum* then actively disables neutrophil bactericidal functions, in particular neutrophil superoxide production, thus promoting its own survival.[64,65] *A phagocytophilum* also reduces neutrophil mobility and phagocytosis,[66] and reduces endothelial adherence and transmigration of neutrophils.[67] By

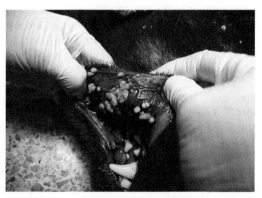

Fig. 4. Viral papillomatosis in a male neutered Rottweiler cross with chronic canine monocytic ehrlichiosis (*From* Ettinger SJ, Feldman EC. Textbook of veterinary internal medicine. 7th edition. St. Louis (MO): Saunders; 2010. Figure 206-1; with permission.)

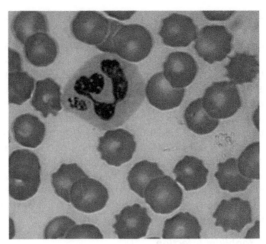

Fig. 5. Morulae of *Anaplasma phagocytophilum* within a canine neutrophil (*From* Ettinger SJ, Feldman EC. Textbook of veterinary internal medicine. 7th edition. St. Louis (MO): Saunders; 2010. Figure 206-2; with permission.)

inhibiting neutrophil apoptosis, the organism is able to survive in a well-differentiated cell that normally has a very short lifespan. The impairment of neutrophil function and leukopenia that develop as a result of *A phagocytophilum* infection is occasionally associated with development of opportunistic infections in some humans and animals with granulocytic anaplasmosis. The best example of this is tick pyemia, which is a debilitating lameness and paralysis that develops in infected lambs in Europe, most commonly as a result of disseminated *Staphylococcus aureus* or *Pasteurella* spp infection. Infection with *A phagocytophilum* may influence the outcome of infection with *Borrelia burgdorferi*, which can be co-transmitted by *Ixodes* ticks, possibly as a result of impaired neutrophil function.[68]

IMMUNOSUPPRESSION CAUSED BY PROTOZOAL AND FUNGAL PATHOGENS

Leishmaniasis, caused by the protozoal parasite *Leishmania infantum*, is a chronic progressive disease transmitted by the sand fly. The mechanisms of immunosuppression induced by this organism are perhaps the best studied amongst protozoal parasites. The disease is most common in the Mediterranean basin and South America. The organism causes a systemic disease in dogs characterized by lymphadenopathy, crusting skin lesions, weight loss, anemia, ocular lesions, polyarthritis, and protein-losing nephropathy. The infection is often associated with other infections, especially ehrlichiosis and babesiosis, and occasionally with neoplastic disease, especially hematopoietic tumors.[69] *Leishmania infantum* invades mononuclear phagocytes, evading the phagolysosome, and survives within them through inhibition of the respiratory burst, inhibition of macrophage function and apoptosis, and impairment of antigen presentation through inhibition of MHC Class I and MHC Class II molecule expression. The protozoan also appears to impair macrophage and neutrophil chemotaxis, and interferes with Il-12 transcription.[70] The *Leishmania* spp surface protein gp63 is a key protein that mediates entry and survival within macrophages. It also allows the organism to resist complement and was recently shown to bind to and suppress the activity of NK cells.[71]

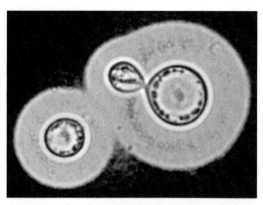

Fig. 6. India ink preparation showing encapsulated yeasts of *Cryptococcus* spp within cerebrospinal fluid. Immunosuppressive properties of the organism have been associated with the glucuronoxylomannan capsule. (*From* Malik M, Krockenberger M, O'Brien CR, et al. Cryptococcosis. In: Greene CE. Infectious diseases of the dog and cat. 3rd edition. St. Louis (MO): Saunders/Elsevier; 2006. p. 584–98. Figure 61-6B; with permission.)

Several fungal pathogens are capable of causing immunosuppression, including *Aspergillus* spp, *Candida* spp, and *Cryptococcus* spp. *Cryptococcus neoformans* and *Cryptococcus gattii* are highly immunosuppressive fungal pathogens, although co-infections with other pathogens are rarely documented. Cryptococcal organisms possess several potent virulence factors that are capable of suppressing or orchestrating the immune response in favor of fungal growth and persistence. The cryptococcal capsular polysaccharide, glucuronoxylomannan, has attracted the most attention in this regard (**Fig. 6**). It effectively inhibits phagocytosis and interferes with migration of leukocytes from the bloodstream into tissues by causing them to shed selectin. It can also deplete complement and directly inhibits T-cell responses.[72,73] There is a shift from a Th1 to a Th2 immune response, the Th1 response being normally required for organism clearance. The cryptococcal urease enzyme was shown to promote accumulation of immature dendritic cells within the lung, and an associated shift in the immune response to a non-protective Th2-cytokine dominated response.[71]

SUMMARY

This review highlights the mechanisms of immunosuppression in just a small subset of the huge variety of infectious agents that are capable of inducing immunosuppression to promote their own survival within the host. The degree of immunosuppression and the mechanisms by which immunodeficiency develops are highly variable and complex. Pathogen surface molecules and cellular receptor tropisms play an important role in determining the initial immune cells infected. Because of the cascading mechanisms involved in normal immune cell recruitment, cytokine and antibody production, pathogens frequently disrupt the function of immune cells that do not undergo direct infection. Considerable research effort has been invested in understanding the mechanisms of pathogen-induced immunosuppression, with the hope that effective therapies may be developed that reverse the immunodeficiencies developed and in turn assist the host to clear persistent or life-threatening infectious diseases.

ACKNOWLEDGMENTS

The authors thank Dr Ellen E. Sparger for her review of the retroviral section of this article.

REFERENCES

1. Beineke A, Puff C, Seehusen F, et al. Pathogenesis and immunopathology of systemic and nervous canine distemper. Vet Immunol Immunopathol 2009; 127(1–2):1–18.
2. Von Messling V, Milosevic D, Cattaneo R. Tropism illuminated: lymphocyte-based pathways blazed by lethal morbillivirus through the host immune system. Proc Natl Acad Sci U S A 2004;101(39):14216–21.
3. Von Messling V, Svitek N, Cattaneo R. Receptor (SLAM [CD150]) recognition and the V protein sustain swift lymphocyte-based invasion of mucosal tissue and lymphatic organs by morbillivirus. J Virol 2006;80(12):6084–92.
4. Appel MJ, Shek WR, Summers BA. Lymphocyte-mediated immune cytotoxicity in dogs infected with virulent canine distemper virus. Infect Immun 1982;37(2): 592–600.
5. Iwatsuki K, Okita M, Ochikubo F, et al. Immunohistochemical analysis of the lymphoid organs of dogs naturally infected with canine distemper virus. J Comp Pathol 1995;113(2):185–90.
6. Wünschmann A, Kremmer E, Baumgärtner W. Phenotypical characterization of T and B cell areas in lymphoid tissues of dogs with spontaneous distemper. Vet Immunol Immunopathol 2000;73(1):83–98.
7. Baumgärtner W, Boyce RW, Alldinger S, et al. Metaphyseal bone lesions in young dogs with systemic canine distemper virus infection. Vet Microbiol 1995;44(2–4): 201–9.
8. Kauffman CA, Bergman AG, O'Connor RP. Distemper virus infection in ferrets: an animal model of measles-induced immunosuppression. Clin Exp Immunol 1982; 47(3):617–25.
9. Wenzlow N, Plattet P, Wittek R, et al. Immunohistochemical demonstration of the putative canine distemper virus receptor CD150 in dogs with and without distemper. Vet Pathol 2007;44(6):943–8.
10. Schobesberger M, Summerfield A, Doherr MG, et al. Canine distemper virus-induced depletion of uninfected lymphocytes is associated with apoptosis. Vet Immunol Immunopathol 2005;104(1–2):33–44.
11. Kerdiles YM, Cherif B, Marie JC, et al. Immunomodulatory properties of morbilli-virus nucleoproteins. Viral Immunol 2006;19(2):324–34.
12. Schneider-Schaulies J, Schneider-Schaulies S. Receptor interactions, tropism, and mechanisms involved in morbillivirus-induced immunomodulation. Adv Virus Res 2008;71:173–205.
13. Ehrensperger F, Pospischil A. [Spontaneous mixed infections with distemper virus and Toxoplasma in dogs]. Dtsch Tierarztl Wochenschr 1989;96(4):184–6 [in German].
14. Smith HW, Buxton A. Incidence of salmonellae in feces of dogs suffering from distemper. Nature 1950;166(4228):824.
15. Fawi MT, Tag el Din MH, el-Sanousi SM. Canine distemper as a predisposing factor for Nocardia asteroides infection in the dog. Vet Rec 1971;88(13):326–8.
16. Ribeiro MG, Salerno T, Mattos-Guaraldi AL, et al. Nocardiosis: an overview and additional report of 28 cases in cattle and dogs. Rev Inst Med Trop Sao Paulo 2008;50(3):177–85.

17. Dyer NW, Schamber GJ. Pneumocystosis associated with canine distemper virus infection in a mink. Can Vet J 1999;40(8):577–8.

18. Lemberger KY, Gondim LF, Pessier AP, et al. *Neospora caninum* infection in a free-ranging raccoon (*Procyon lotor*) with concurrent canine distemper virus infection. J Parasitol 2005;91(4):960–1.

19. Lamm CG, Rezabek GB. Parvovirus infection in domestic companion animals. Vet Clin North Am Small Anim Pract 2008;38(4):837–50, viii-ix.

20. Hueffer K, Parrish CR. Parvovirus host range, cell tropism and evolution. Curr Opin Microbiol 2003;6(4):392–8.

21. Pollock RV. Experimental canine parvovirus infection in dogs. Cornell Vet 1982; 72(2):103–19.

22. Krakowka S, Olsen RG, Axthelm MK, et al. Canine parvovirus infection potentiates canine distemper encephalitis attributable to modified live-virus vaccine. J Am Vet Med Assoc 1982;180(2):137–9.

23. Carlson JH, Scott FW, Duncan JR. Feline Panleukopenia. I. Pathogenesis in germfree and specific pathogen-free cats. Vet Pathol 1977;14(1):79–88.

24. Mendoza R, Anderson MM, Overbaugh J. A putative thiamine transport protein is a receptor for feline leukemia virus subgroup A. J Virol 2006;80(7):3378–85.

25. Anderson MM, Lauring AS, Robertson S. Feline Pit2 functions as a receptor for subgroup B feline leukemia viruses. J Virol 2001;75(22):10563–72.

26. Keel SB, Doty RT, Yang Z, et al. A heme export protein is required for red blood cell differentiation and iron homeostasis. Science 2008;319(5864):825–8.

27. Anderson MM, Lauring AS, Burns CC, et al. Identification of a cellular cofactor required for infection by feline leukemia virus. Science 2000;287(5459): 1828–30.

28. Kipar A, Kremendahl J, Grant CK, et al. Expression of viral proteins in feline leukemia virus-associated enteritis. Vet Pathol 2000;37(2):129–36.

29. Good RA, Ogasawara M, Liu WT, et al. Immunosuppressive actions of retroviruses. Lymphology 1990;23(2):56–9.

30. Cianciolo GJ, Copeland TD, Oroszlan S, et al. Inhibition of lymphocyte proliferation by a synthetic peptide homologous to retroviral envelope proteins. Science 1985;230(4724):453–5.

31. Mitani M, Cianciolo GJ, Snyderman R, et al. Suppressive effect on polyclonal B-cell activation of a synthetic peptide homologous to a transmembrane component of oncogenic retroviruses. Proc Natl Acad Sci U S A 1987;84(1):237–40.

32. Haraguchi S, Good RA, Day-Good NK. A potent immunosuppressive retroviral peptide: cytokine patterns and signaling pathways. Immunol Res 2008;41(1): 46–55.

33. Cockerell GL, Hoover EA, Krakowka S, et al. Lymphocyte mitogen reactivity and enumeration of circulating B- and T-cells during feline leukemia virus infection in the cat. J Natl Cancer Inst 1976;57(5):1095–9.

34. Hebebrand LC, Mathes LE, Olsen RG. Inhibition of concanavalin A stimulation of feline lymphocytes by inactivated feline leukemia virus. Cancer Res 1977;37(12): 4532–3.

35. Mathes LE, Olsen RG, Hebebrand LC, et al. Abrogation of lymphocyte blastogenesis by a feline leukaemia virus protein. Nature 1978;274(5672):687–9.

36. Perryman LE, Hoover EA, Yohn DS. Immunologic reactivity of the cat: immunosuppression in experimental feline leukemia. J Natl Cancer Inst 1972;49(5): 1357–65.

37. Trainin Z, Wernicke D, Ungar-Waron H, et al. Suppression of the humoral antibody response in natural retrovirus infections. Science 1983;220(4599):858–9.

38. Wernicke D, Trainin Z, Ungar-Waron H, et al. Humoral immune response of asymptomatic cats naturally infected with feline leukemia virus. J Virol 1986; 60(2):669–73.

39. Lafrado LJ, Olsen RG. Demonstration of depressed polymorphonuclear leukocyte function in nonviremic FeLV-infected cats. Cancer Invest 1986;4(4):297–300.

40. Hoffmann-Jagielska M, Winnicka A, Jagielski D, et al. Influence of naturally acquired feline leukemia virus (FeLV) infection on the phagocytic and respiratory burst activity of neutrophils and monocytes of peripheral blood. Pol J Vet Sci 2005;8(2):93–7.

41. Wardini AB, Guimarães-Costa AB, Nascimento MT, et al. Characterization of neutrophil extracellular traps in cats naturally infected with feline leukemia virus. J Gen Virol 2010;91(Pt 1):259–64.

42. Sykes JE, Malik R. Cryptococcosis. In: Greene CE, editor. Infectious diseases of the dog and cat. 4th edition. St Louis (MO): Saunders Elsevier, in press.

43. de Parseval A, Chatterji U, Sun P, et al. Feline immunodeficiency virus targets activated CD4+ T cells by using CD134 as a binding receptor. Proc Natl Acad Sci U S A 2004;101(35):13044–9.

44. Shimojima M, Miyazawa T, Ikeda Y, et al. Use of CD134 as a primary receptor by the feline immunodeficiency virus. Science 2004;303(5661):1192–5.

45. Tompkins MB, Tompkins WA. Lentivirus-induced immune dysregulation. Vet Immunol Immunopathol 2008;123(1–2):45–55.

46. Yamamoto JK, Sparger E, Ho EW, et al. Pathogenesis of experimentally induced feline immunodeficiency virus infection in cats. Am J Vet Res 1988;49(8): 1246–58.

47. Sprague WS, Terwee JA, Vandewoude S. Temporal association of large granular lymphocytosis, neutropenia, proviral load, and FasL mRNA in cats with acute feline immunodeficiency virus infection. Vet Immunol Immunopathol 2010; 134(1–2):115–21.

48. Mexas AM, Fogle JE, Tompkins WA, et al. CD4+CD25+ regulatory T cells are infected and activated during acute FIV infection. Vet Immunol Immunopathol 2008;126(3–4):263–72.

49. Vahlenkamp TW, Tompkins MB, Tompkins WA. Feline immunodeficiency virus infection phenotypically and functionally activates immunosuppressive CD4+CD25+ T regulatory cells. J Immunol 2004;172(8):4752–61.

50. Dean GA, LaVoy A, Yearley J, et al. Cytokine modulation of the innate immune response in feline immunodeficiency virus-infected cats. J Infect Dis 2006; 193(11):1520–7.

51. Lehman TL, O'Halloran KP, Hoover EA, et al. Utilizing the FIV model to understand dendritic cell dysfunction and the potential role of dendritic cell immunization in HIV infection. Vet Immunol Immunopathol 2010;134(1–2):75–81.

52. Levy JK, Liang Y, Ritchey JW, et al. Failure of FIV-infected cats to control Toxoplasma gondii correlates with reduced IL2, IL6, and IL12 and elevated IL10 expression by lymph node T cells. Vet Immunol Immunopathol 2004;98(1–2):101–11.

53. de Groot-Mijnes JD, van Dun JM, van der Most RG, et al. Natural history of a recurrent feline coronavirus infection and the role of cellular immunity in survival and disease. J Virol 2005;79(2):1036–44.

54. Weinman D. Human bartonella infection and African sleeping sickness. Bull N Y Acad Med 1946;22(12):647–70.

55. Pappalado BL, Brown T, Gebhardt D, et al. Cyclic CD8+ lymphopenia in dogs infected with Bartonella vinsonii subspecies berkhoffii. Vet Immunol Immunopathol 2000;75(1–2):43–57.

56. Baker HJ, Cassell GH, Lindsey JR. Research complications due to *Haemobarto-nella* and *Eperythrozoon* infections in experimental animals. Am J Pathol 1971; 64(3):625–32.
57. Philbey AW, Barron RC, Gounden A. Chronic eperythrozoonosis in an adult ewe. Vet Rec 2006;158:662–4.
58. Breitschwerdt EB, Woody BJ, Zerbe CA, et al. Monoclonal gammopathy associ-ated with naturally occurring canine ehrlichiosis. J Vet Intern Med 1987;1(1):2–9.
59. Schroeder H, Jardine JE, Davis V. Systemic phaeohyphomycosis caused by *Xy-lohypha bantiana* in a dog. J S Afr Vet Assoc 1994;65(4):175–8.
60. Mekuzas Y, Gradoni L, Oliva G, et al. *Ehrlichia canis* and *Leishmania infantum* co-infection: a 3-year longitudinal study in naturally exposed dogs. Clin Microbiol Infect 2009. [Epub ahead of print].
61. Harrus S, Waner T, Friedmann-Morvinski D, et al. Down-regulation of MHC class II receptors of DH82 cells, following infection with *Ehrlichia canis*. Vet Immunol Im-munopathol 2003;96(3–4):239–43.
62. Hess PR, English RV, Hegarty BC, et al. Experimental *Ehrlichia canis* infection in the dog does not cause immunosuppression. Vet Immunol Immunopathol 2006; 109(1–2):117–25.
63. Carrade DD, Foley JE, Borjesson DL, et al. Canine granulocytic anaplasmosis – a review. J Vet Intern Med 2009;23(6):1129–41.
64. Rikihisa Y. *Ehrlichia* subversion of host innate responses. Curr Opin Microbiol 2006;9:95–101.
65. Carlyon JA, Fikrig E. Mechanism of evasion of neutrophil killing by *Anaplasma phagocytophilum*. Curr Opin Hematol 2006;13:28–33.
66. Garyu JW, Choi KS, Grab DJ, et al. Defective phagocytosis in *Anaplasma phag-ocytophilum* infected neutrophils. Infect Immun 2005;73:1187–90.
67. Choi KS, Garyu J, Park J, et al. Diminished adhesion of *Anaplasma phagocyto-philum*-infected neutrophils to endothelial cells is associated with reduced expression of leukocyte surface selectin. Infect Immun 2003;71:4586–94.
68. Nyarko E, Grab DJ, Dumler JS. *Anaplasma phagocytophilum*-infected neutro-phils enhance transmigration of *Borrelia burgdorferi* across the human blood brain barrier in vitro. Int J Parasitol 2006;36:601–5.
69. Foglia Manzillo V, Pagano A, Guglielmino R, et al. Extranodal gammadelta-T-cell lymphoma in a dog with leishmaniasis. Vet Clin Pathol 2008;37(3):298–301.
70. Zambrano-Villa S, Rosales-Borjas D, Carrero JC, et al. How protozoan parasites evade the host immune response. Trends Parasitol 2002;18(6):272–8.
71. Lieke T, Nylén S, Eidsmo L, et al. *Leishmania* surface protein gp63 binds directly to human natural killer cells and inhibits proliferation. Clin Exp Immunol 2008; 153(2):221–30.
72. Yauch LE, Lam JS, Levitz SM. Direct inhibition of T-cell responses by the *Crypto-coccus* capsular polysaccharide glucuronoxylomannan. PLoS Pathog 2006; 2(11):e120.
73. Osterholzer JJ, Surana R, Milam JE, et al. Cryptococcal urease promotes the accumulation of immature dendritic cells and a non-protective T2 immune response within the lung. Am J Pathol 2009;174(3):932–43.

Primary Immunodeficiencies of Dogs and Cats

Mary C. DeBey, DVM, PhD

KEYWORDS

- Immunodeficiency • Hypogammaglobulinemia
- Anomaly • Syndrome • Recurrent infection

Primary immunodeficiencies are congenital defects that affect formation or function of cells or proteins of the immune system. There are doubtless many immunodeficiencies of dogs and cats that have not been identified. Some human immunologists estimate that approximately 1 in 500 babies born in the United States has a defect in the immune system.[1] It is likely that many immune defects in dogs and cats are not severe enough to be life threatening. Defects may occur in neutrophils, lymphocytes, or other components of the innate or adaptive immune system. As veterinarians become more aware of congenital immune disease in pets, more syndromes will be identified.

Veterinarians are faced with identifying pets that have immune compromise and with the guiding care of those animals. Repeated infections in a young animal, usually after weaning or loss of maternal immunoglobulins, may indicate congenital immunodeficiency. Several defects of neutrophils have been described that may result in abnormal appearance, formation, release, or function. Defects of lymphocytes usually occur during formation and affect the cell-mediated or humoral arm of the immune system. Historically, most primary immunodeficiency disorders are recognized in purebred puppies and are breed related. Fewer problems have been identified in kittens. With appropriate antimicrobial treatment, lifespan can often be extended.[2]

Diagnosis of immunodeficiency may include routine complete blood count, with special attention to the leukogram, total protein, and globulin level. In some cases a bone marrow aspirate is indicated. Commercial kits (Diagnostic Laboratory, College of Veterinary Medicine, Cornell University, Ithaca, NY, USA, www.vet.cornell.edu) are available to measure IgG, IgM, and IgA levels in serum. Most lymphocyte and neutrophil function assays are limited to research laboratories.[3]

A full necropsy is indicated for any deceased animal with suspected primary immunodeficiency. During the necropsy, all lymphoid organs should be evaluated.

Hill's Veterinary Consultation Service, Hill's Pet Nutrition, Inc, 400 SW 8th Avenue, Topeka, KS, USA
E-mail address: marydebey@networksplus.net

Vet Clin Small Anim 40 (2010) 425–438
doi:10.1016/j.cvsm.2010.01.001
0195-5616/10/$ – see front matter

Appropriate samples of thymus, spleen, lymph node, bone marrow, and intestine should be collected for histopathology.[3]

INHERITED DEFICIENCIES OF NEUTROPHILS
Defective Formation of Neutrophils

Pelger-Huët anomaly

Neutrophils in pets with the Pelger-Huët anomaly have rounded nuclei and fail to lobulate as they mature. Pets affected with this condition are frequently healthy, with no history of repeated infections that are often associated with primary immunodeficiencies.[2]

Diagnosis of Pelger-Huët may be an incidental finding during routine examination of a blood smear during a wellness examination. A dog or cat may have no sign of systemic disease. Nevertheless, the blood smear from an individual with Pelger-Huët has many neutrophils that appear to be immature because there is no segmenting of the nucleus. Close examination of the neutrophils reveals condensed nuclear chromatin, indicating that the cells are mature.[4]

Pelger-Huët anomaly has been reported in cocker spaniels, basenjis, Boston terriers, foxhounds, coonhounds, Australian shepherds, and domestic shorthair cats.[2] Pelger-Huët neutrophils may be less able to migrate to affected areas because of suspected inflexible nuclei. Some studies have reported possible inhibition of B-cell response to antigen.[4] The Pelger-Huët anomaly, however, seems to have little effect on the life and health of animals.[2]

Canine leukocyte adhesion deficiency

For neutrophils to get to an area of inflammation, they must adhere to proteins on endothelial cells that have been stimulated by local inflammation. The proteins involved in adherence of neutrophils to endothelial cells are called integrins (on the neutrophil) and selectins (on the blood vessel wall).[5] The integrin molecule on the neutrophil has two components—CD11b and CD18—which associate with each other before they are expressed as the integrin on the neutrophil surface. Neutrophils from dogs affected with canine leukocyte adherence deficiency (CLAD) do not express the integrin on their cell surface and consequently cannot stick to endothelial cells. Therefore, neutrophils are not able to get to the area of inflammation, and bacteria in tissues can survive and multiply more readily. Neutrophils from CLAD dogs fail to adhere normally to plastic surfaces and are unable to ingest particles opsonized with C3b.[6]

Affected puppies may have partial or complete deficiency of the integrin. Deficiency of the integrin causes puppies to present with recurrent infections. Puppies with partial deficiencies have less severe clinical signs than puppies with a complete deficiency of the integrin. The most striking feature of the disease alerting the primary care veterinarian of the problem is an extraordinarily high white blood cell count with a profound left shift.[2] Puppies may also have severe gingivitis and superficial dermatitis or fistulas.[7]

CLAD has been described in Irish setters and in a related breed, the Irish red and white setter.[7] The disease is likely carried as an autosomal recessive. Asymptomatic carriers maintain the defect in the population. The mutation site is in the CD18 portion of the integrin of Irish red and white setters. In the United Kingdom, a commercial diagnostic test to check for carriers in Irish red and white setters is reported.[8] Testing has been discontinued in Australia because selective breeding of tested dogs has resulted in low incidence of the allele.[9]

Puppies affected with CLAD have been successfully treated with bone marrow transplantation.[10] If the transplantation was performed before 4 months of age, the puppies went on to reproduce with no more complications than CLAD carriers.[11]

Chédiak-Higashi syndrome

Chédiak-Higashi syndrome is considered an autosomal recessive disorder of cats that manifests as hypopigmentation of eyes and hair.[12,13] No cases have been reported in dogs. The syndrome has been described specifically in Persian cats with blue smoke hair color. Affected cats had blue and cream or blue smoke hair color and yellow eyes, whereas unaffected cats had copper colored eyes.[13,14] Cats exhibit photophobia and may develop cataracts. After intentional rotation during a physical examination, they may exhibit prolonged nystagmus.[12] Recurrent infections and decreased bactericidal function of neutrophils in affected animals have been reported.[2] Loss of tapetal pigmentation and normal rod structure progresses with age. At 14 days of age, the eyes appear normal, but by 28 days of age, loss of tapetum has been documented. After 1 year of age, the tapetal layer is essentially gone.[13]

On a blood smear, the neutrophils have large intracytoplasmic vesicles, described as lysosomes. The granules vary in size from the limit of resolution of the light microscope to slightly greater than 2 μm.[14] Intracytoplasmic granules may occur in other cell types. Enlarged melanin granules are present in hair.[2,15] If a cat has enlarged melanin granules in hair and in neutrophils, the diagnosis is likely Chédiak-Higashi syndrome.

Neutropenia is observed in cats affected with Chédiak-Higashi syndrome.[16] Treatment of affected cats in one previous study demonstrated that canine granulocyte colony-stimulating factor restored neutrophil numbers, migratory ability, and phagocytosis.[17] The currently accepted treatment, however, is a bone marrow transplant.

Canine cyclic hematopoiesis

Canine cyclic hematopoiesis, also known as gray collie syndrome or cyclic neutropenia, is a disease in collies characterized by muted hair color and cyclic neutropenic episodes.[2] Intermittent hypoplasia of bone marrow also occurs.[18] Previous studies demonstrated a cycle takes place every 11 to 13 days. Profound neutropenia precedes a transient neutrophilia followed by a mild decrease in neutrophils, then a second neutrophilia followed by profound neutropenia.[18] Throughout the cycle, neutrophils from affected dogs display defective ability to kill ingested bacteria.[19]

The condition is inherited as an autosomal recessive. Affected dogs present with dilution of skin pigmentation and recurrent respiratory or gastrointestinal infections. Puppies may exhibit delayed wound healing, stunted growth, and high mortality, especially after loss of maternal immunity.[2] Neutrophil counts may go below 500/μL during the cycle. Eosinophils increase during the neutropenic episodes. Absolute numbers of monocytes, reticulocytes, and platelets also fluctuate during the cycle but do not correspond with neutrophil numbers, probably due to differences in maturation times in the bone marrow.[18] Downward fluctuations in platelet counts may lead to bleeding problems. Chronic infections occur, particularly during the neutropenic period.[2]

Cyclic hematopoiesis has been corrected experimentally with appropriate bone marrow transplant/grafting.[20] Defective marrow stem cells are likely the cause of the cyclic neutropenia, because cyclic hematopoiesis was transmitted to normal dogs by transplantation of gray collie marrow.[21] Lithium carbonate and endotoxin can stabilize production of blood cells, including neutrophils, but both are toxic with repeated injections.[2] Neither treatment permanently corrects the condition. The prognosis is poor. Most affected dogs do not live past 3 years of age.[2]

Trapped neutrophil syndrome

Trapped neutrophil syndrome seems to be a condition distinct from cyclic hematopoiesis and is inherited as an autosomal recessive.[22] The defect is not carried in the same gene as a similar syndrome in humans, and genetic analysis indicates trapped neutrophil syndrome is not the same as cyclic hematopoiesis.[23,24] Although cases first described in the literature occurred in border collies in Australia and New Zealand, border collies in many countries are carriers of the defect.[25] Affected dogs present with history and signalment similar to dogs with cyclic hematopoiesis. Bone marrow aspirates, however, are hypercellular with primarily myeloid cells, in contrast to the occasional hypocellular appearance of bone marrow of cyclic hematopoiesis. Neutropenia appears concurrently with bone marrow myeloid hyperplasia.[22] Most affected puppies die or are euthanized by 4 months of age. Genetic testing is available to detect carriers.[25]

Granulocyte colony-stimulating factor deficiency in a rottweiler

A 3-year-old male rottweiler presented with fever, shifting leg lameness (arthritis), enlarged lymph nodes, conjunctivitis, otitis, persistent neutropenia, and elevated globulins. A bone marrow aspirate revealed incomplete maturation of granulocytes. Treatment with antibiotics gave only temporary relief of clinical signs. Testing revealed a deficiency of granulocyte colony-stimulating factor as a cause of the chronic neutropenia. Treatment with human recombinant granulocyte colony-stimulating factor was declined for financial reasons and because of concern about development of antibodies to the protein with chronic treatment. No mode of inheritance was determined.[26]

Defective Neutrophil Function

Canine granulocytopathy syndrome of Irish setters

Puppies from a colony of Irish setters were more susceptible to infection than randomly bred controls. Deficient bactericidal activity was due to inability of neutrophils to generate a respiratory burst because of a defective hexose monophosphate shunt. The defect was inherited as an autosomal recessive, and male and female dogs were affected. The affected dogs were more susceptible to pyogenic infections and had shorter life spans than controls. Omphalophlebitis, gingivitis, lymphadenopathy, suppurative skin lesions, and osteomyelitis were observed.[27] The described disease was similar to CLAD with a persistent neutrophilia and left shift. Canine granulocytopathy syndrome may be a variant of CLAD or may be a separate syndrome caused by defective bactericidal activity.[2]

Weimaraners

Defective neutrophil function has been reported in weimaraners.[28,29] Urate crystals were observed in the urine of some weimaraners with granulocytosis or defective neutrophil function.[29,30] Increased turnover of nucleoprotein from catabolism of spent neutrophils was postulated as the cause of the urate crystalluria, because there was no diagnosis of liver disease.[29,30] No testing was reported to rule out portosystemic shunt, however, as a reason for the urate crystalluria. Low IgG was present in dogs with neutrophil dysfunction, and is discussed under immunoglobulin deficiencies.

Doberman pinschers

Closely related Doberman pinschers presented with chronic rhinitis and pneumonia. The dogs had dull haircoats with seborrhea and scaling. The hemogram was normal in about half the dogs. Neutrophilia without a left shift occurred in three of the eight dogs tested. Four of the dogs had bronchopneumonia radiographically, and four did not (the four without bronchopneumonia had cardiomyopathy). Concentrations of immunoglobulin were normal or increased, and lymphocyte function tests were not consistently different from controls. Neutrophils had a defect in killing. Recurrent infections responded to antibiotics.[31]

DEFECTS OF LYMPHOCYTES
Severe Combined Immunodeficiency and X-linked Severe Combined Immunodeficiency

Severe combined immunodeficiency (SCID) and X-linked SCID (XSCID) have been reported in dogs. SCID, in which lymphocyte development is blocked at the prolymphocyte stage, results in profound deficiency of B and T lymphocytes. It has been reported in Jack Russell terriers.[32] The defect occurs during genetic recombination (V[D]J recombination), which is essential for formation of the antigen recognition site of lymphocytes. SCID in Jack Russell terriers is similar to the disease in Arabian foals, but blocking of recombination is not as complete as in SCID foals. Affected puppies died of opportunistic infections within 8 to 14 weeks of age.[32]

XSCID has been reported in Cardigan Welsh corgis and basset hounds and affects only male puppies. XSCID puppies may not be profoundly lymphopenic as are SCID puppies. Lymphocyte numbers, however, are reduced. Most of the lymphocytes are B cells (cells potentially capable of producing immunoglobulins). IgM is present but IgG and IgA levels are low or nonexistent, and the puppies are hypogammaglobulinemic.[2,33,34]

Puppies with XSCID usually present after weaning with a history of failure to thrive. They appear stunted compared with their normal littermates.[33] During physical examination, peripheral lymph nodes are not palpable, and no tonsils are visible. Diarrhea, vomiting, respiratory infection, and superficial pyoderma are commonly reported because of increased susceptibility to viral and bacterial diseases.[2,33] XSCID dogs that were vaccinated with modified live distemper virus vaccine died of vaccine-induced distemper. XSCID puppies die by 3 to 4 months of age, often of generalized staphylococcal infections.[33]

Bone marrow transplantation has been used successfully in XSCID dogs at 2 to 3 weeks of age. T cells were evident in 30 days,[34–36] and IgG levels reached normal levels after 4 to 6 months.[35] Unfortunately, 70% of transplanted dogs developed interdigital or footpad papillomas within 1 to 2 years of age. Most papillomas did not regress spontaneously and were painful, and some progressed to squamous cell carcinomas. Several dogs were euthanized because of painful lameness due to the papillomas. The lack of a mononuclear infiltrate in biopsies of papillomas from XCID dogs has led to speculation about Langerhans cell dysfunction in the skin.[37]

Suspected Combined Immunodeficiency Syndrome in Rottweilers

A litter of eight rottweiler puppies was investigated for primary congenital immunodeficiency disease because two of the puppies died of systemic disease before 6 months of age, another puppy contracted systemic demodecosis, and a fourth puppy had persistent subcutaneous abscesses.[38] Postmortem examination of lymphoid tissues from the deceased puppies revealed a few T lymphocytes and follicles with B lymphocytes. Plasma cells were absent from some lymphoid tissues, however. All the puppies in the litter had normal IgM and abnormally low IgA. Seven of the eight puppies had low IgG. The immunoglobulin levels were similar to those reported for immunodeficient weimeraners.[39] In addition, other related rottweilers also had low IgA levels. Irregular maturation of B-cell lymphocytes to plasma cells and lack of class switching were evident. The investigators theorized that lack of cytokine signals from T-cell lymphocytes might be the underlying defect, making this a form of combined immunodeficiency.[38] Four of the puppies were clinically normal even though they had low levels of IgA immunoglobulin, lending support to the speculation that carriers of an immunodeficiency survive in the breed. Pedigrees were not revealed.

Hypotrichosis with Thymic Aplasia in Birman Kittens

Birman kittens were presented because they were hairless. Hairless kittens from some litters were born dead or died shortly after birth. Some of the hairless kittens grew normally and were active until the owner requested euthanasia. No therapy was attempted for these kittens. None of the hairless kittens lived beyond 13 weeks of age. All of the parents of affected kittens had a common great-great-grandsire. The condition is most likely inherited as an autosomal recessive.[40]

At necropsy, no thymus was grossly visible. Histologically, there was no thymus parenchyma or Hassall corpuscles in the normal location for the thymus. Lymph nodes and spleen appeared normal at gross necropsy. Histologic examination, however, revealed the paracortical (T-cell dependent) regions of lymphoid tissue were depleted of lymphocytes.[40] Therefore, these kittens were deficient in T lymphocytes.[2]

Primary hair follicles and sweat glands in the skin were decreased in number and hypoplastic when compared with normal, age-matched kittens. No hairs were observed in the hair follicles. Sebaceous glands, however, were normal.[40]

Hypotrichosis indicates a failure of normal development of ectoderm, whereas thymic aplasia represents an anomaly of endodermal development. The presence of ectodermal and endodermal anomalies makes any potential future therapy challenging.

Suppressed Cell-mediated Cutaneous Immunity in Young Doberman Pinschers

A Doberman kennel had a recurring problem with generalized demodicosis in puppies over 12 weeks of age. Healthy, related Doberman puppies from the kennel demonstrated suppressed cutaneous cell-mediated immunity. Adult dogs from the kennel had normal cutaneous reactions, which indicated the defect was age related. The investigators suggested that defective cutaneous cell-mediated immunity in these puppies was heritable, were age related, and contributed to the prevalence of generalized demodecosis.[41]

Lethal Acrodermatitis in Bull Terriers

Lethal acrodermatitis is an inherited autosomal recessive. Affected puppies are born with lighter pigmentation than unaffected littermates. Lymph nodes may be small. At weaning, affected puppies are smaller than their littermates and have difficulty eating. Food gets lodged in the high arch of the hard palate. The feet become splayed and interdigital, crusted lesions appear at 6 to 10 weeks. Crusted lesions with high numbers of Malassezia and Candida also appear at the mucocutaneous junctions.[42] Affected puppies have chronic or intermittent diarrhea and respiratory tract infections. Infections may be refractory to treatment. The median survival time is 7 months.[43–45] Zinc supplementation does not correct the disorder.[43,45] Measurement of zinc levels is not helpful for diagnosis. The presence of splayed feet and skin lesions on the face and feet are helpful, however, in identifying affected individuals. Research has demonstrated that B- and T-lymphocyte function is decreased in lymphocyte assays, and IgA levels are low.[43,46] Some investigators speculate that lethal acrodermatitis in bull terriers may be a combined immunodeficiency disease.[46]

Growth Hormone Deficiency in Weimaraners

A syndrome described in Weimaraner puppies caused wasting, emaciation, lethargy, and persistent infections leading to death after a few weeks of age. The thymic cortex was absent and lymphocyte reactions to mitogens were deficient. After treatment with growth hormone, the thymus increased in size and cellularity. Lymphocyte response to mitogens remained deficient, however. Growth hormone was administered at 0.1 mg/kg subcutaneously daily for 5 days, then on alternate days for five doses, then every 3 days for four additional doses. The dogs responded to treatment. The wasting syndrome was reversed, their appetite was improved, and the dogs remained clinically normal 2 to 4 years later.[47]

Rhinitis/Bronchopneumonia Syndrome in the Irish Wolfhound

Rhinitis/bronchopneumonia syndrome in the Irish wolfhound is characterized by serous to mucopurulent, intermittent to persistent nasal discharge, frequently accompanied by bronchopneumonia. Affected dogs are related, indicating that the syndrome is due to an inherited immunodeficiency.[48,49] *Pasteurella*, *Klebsiella*, *Mycoplasma*, *Staphylococcus*, and *Streptococcus* spp as well as *Escherichia coli* have been cultured from the exudates.

Evidence indicates some affected dogs have mild defects of nasal or bronchial cilia, observed by electron microscopy.[49] The changes were not as severe as those recognized in primary ciliary dyskinesia. Histopathology of peripheral lymph nodes may reveal depleted parafollicular areas, indicating a possible T-cell disorder.[48] Globulin levels are normal in most affected dogs. Immunoglobulin levels were lower during acute episodes in some dogs, however, leading to speculation of a cyclic defect in immunoglobulin concentrations.[49]

Affected dogs often live several years into adulthood if the pneumonia continues to respond to antibiotics. Owners should be warned about recurrence of intractable mucoid nasal discharge and possible pneumonia throughout a dog's life.

COMPLEMENT DEFICIENCY

Brittany spaniel dogs with C3 deficiency exhibited recurrent sepsis, pneumonia, pyometra, and wound infections. Dogs that were carriers had about half the normal levels of C3 and were clinically normal. Homozygous individuals had no detectable C3. Some affected dogs developed glomerulonephritis, leading to kidney failure.[50,51] Dogs with deficiencies of other complement factors are probably asymptomatic, because humans and pigs with deficiencies of complement components other than C3 are clinically normal.[51]

IMMUNOGLOBULIN DISORDERS

Immunoglobulin deficiencies occur in many dog breeds. The exact genetic cause of various immunoglobulin deficiencies is unknown in many cases. A defect in T-helper cell function, cytokine signaling, or failure to switch classes of immunoglobulin during B-cell maturation are all possible mechanisms leading to immunoglobulin deficiencies. The net result is low or absent IgM, IgG, or IgA on mucosal surfaces or in serum. In general, dogs with deficiency of only one class of immunoglobulin have milder clinical signs than those with deficiency of more than 1 class. Reference laboratories (Diagnostic Laboratory, College of Veterinary Medicine, Cornell University, Ithaca, NY 14853-6401, USA, www.vet.cornell.edu) have kits available to measure levels of serum IgM, IgG, or IgA to identify and diagnose deficiencies. Infections should be treated with appropriate antimicrobials. There is no cure at this time.

IMMUNODEFICIENCIES ASSOCIATED WITH *PNEUMOCYSTIS CARINII*
Miniature Dachshunds

Common variable immunodeficiency, in which B lymphocytes produce little or no antibody, has been reported in miniature dachshunds.[52] The history includes repeated infections in a young patient, usually less than 1 year of age, and treated successfully with antibiotics. Recurrent infections—enteritis, tonsillitis, dermatitis, and otitis—are common. Lymphocyte count may be elevated, normal, or decreased.[52] Globulins were frequently low or low normal, despite chronic infections.[52–54] Lymphocyte function assays demonstrated an inability to proliferate normally.[52,53]

Symptomatic treatment of infections with antibiotics was successful, but the infections recurred. Puppies described in the literature presented tachypnic because of infection with *Pneumocystis carinii*. The infection was diagnosed with tracheal wash cytology or at necropsy. The most common treatment of *P carinii* is with trimethoprim/sulfamethoxazole (15 mg/kg 3 times a day or 30 mg/kg twice a day for 3 to 6 weeks).[54,55] Long-term prognosis is guarded.

Cavalier King Charles Spaniels

A syndrome in cavalier King Charles spaniels has been described in which the dogs have increased susceptibility to *P carinii*.[55–57] The median age at presentation with pneumocystis pneumonia is 3.5 years. Tachypnea, absence of fever, leukocytosis, and atrophic or nonpalpable lymph nodes are common findings on physical examination.[55,56] Globulins may be normal or elevated. When serum electrophoresis is performed, however, there is hypogammaglobulinemia, indicating a defect in humoral immunity. IgM is normal or high and IgG is low; there is apparently a defect in the ability of B cells to switch from IgM to IgG.[55,57] Investigators speculate about, but have never tested for, a cell-mediated defect similar to the combined variable immunodeficiency of miniature dachshunds. The immune defects are different, however, because miniature dachshunds present with pneumocystis pneumonia before 1 year of age, and cavalier King Charles spaniels are usually over 1 year of age. *P carinii* is treated with 3 to 6 weeks of trimethoprim/sulfamethoxazole.

Other Breeds

Pneumocystis pneumonia has been described in a 14-month-old male Yorkshire terrier that received long-term prednisone for tracheobronchitis.[58] Immunodeficiency was suspected because clinical signs associated with the pneumonia occurred before 1 year of age. Neutropenia and lymphopenia were reported. The investigators, however, were unable to rule out the long-term steroid therapy as a contributing factor in the fatal pneumocystis pneumonia.[58]

A 1-year-old beagle demonstrated compromised cell-mediated immunity, which was confirmed with an intradermal test.[59] The dog died with generalized demodicosis. *P carinii* pneumonia was diagnosed at necropsy. Suppressed cell-mediated immunity associated with *Demodex canis* and *P carinii* led the investigators to speculate that a heritable immunodeficiency was present.[59]

DEFICIENCIES OF A PRIMARY CLASS OF IMMUNOGLOBULINS
IgM Deficiency—Doberman Pinschers

IgM deficiency was described in young Doberman pinschers. One puppy with IgM deficiency only, and normal levels of IgG and IgA, was clinically normal. A related puppy with low IgM and low IgG had persistent nasal discharge and pneumonia, which responded to antibiotic therapy. Clinical signs returned each time antibiotics were discontinued. The dog was successfully treated with daily antibiotics for life.[60]

IgG Deficiency—Weimaraners

Immunodeficiency in Weimaraners is characterized by recurrent infections and hypo-gammaglobulinemia.[28,29,39,61–63] IgG is frequently the only immunoglobulin class that is low.[28,29,62,63] Low IgA along with low IgG has been reported, however.[39] In one report about a litter of Weimaraner puppies, only 2 of 10 puppies produced protective antibodies to parvovirus.[62] Vaccination with parvovirus vaccine only, followed by distemper vaccine without parvovirus 2 weeks later, may be beneficial for immune response in some puppies.[62] Foods with a single source of protein were helpful in some cases of enteritis.[63]

IgA Deficiency

Immunodeficiency due to low levels of IgA is common in dogs.[64] IgG or IgM deficiency may be present along with IgA deficiency.[64] Prevalence in the canine population at large is unknown, because deficiency of IgA is not always associated with clinical disease. Other immunoglobulin classes sometimes compensate for the lack of IgA,[64–66] and the affected dog remains clinically normal. A high incidence of IgA deficiency has been detected in shar-peis,[64,67,68] beagles,[64,69] dachshunds, Dalmatians, Akitas, chows, West Highland white terriers, miniature schnauzers, cocker spaniels,[64] German shepherds,[64,66,70–74] and mixed breed dogs.[64] IgA deficiency has also been reported in Irish setters,[64,75] Dobermans, golden retrievers, and poodles.[64] Low IgA levels in serum have been reported in at least one dog from several other breeds—Yorkshire terrier, Welsh corgi, Newfoundland, Irish wolfhound, soft-coated wheaten terrier, Old English sheepdog, cairn terrier, and keeshond.[64] Dogs with IgA deficiency may present with pyoderma,[64,68] atopy, otitis,[64] demodecosis[64,67] chronic bronchitis,[64,69] recurrent pneumonia[67,75] food allergy,[64] or enteritis.[69–72,74,76]

Serum IgA levels to determine deficiency should not be assessed before 16 weeks of age, because normal puppies may have low IgA before that age.[67] IgA concentrations were low in normal shar-pei puppies when they were 4 to 10 weeks of age.[67] Any dog with selective IgA deficiency or a chronic or recurring skin problem should not be used for breeding.[68]

In dogs, almost all serum IgA is dimeric and comes from plasma cells in respiratory, conjunctival, reproductive, and intestinal mucosa.[65,71] Most serum IgA likely comes from intestinal mucosa[71] because it is the largest mucosal surface. Low concentrations of serum IgA may or may not correlate with higher secreted IgA, for instance in tears.[65,73]

Small intestinal bacterial overgrowth (SIBO), defined as greater than 10^5 bacteria per mL of duodenal juice, has been associated with IgA deficiency.[70,71,76,77] Enteric bacteria can synthesize folate and many can bind cobalamin (vitamin B12) within the lumen. Therefore, SIBO may or may not be accompanied by elevated folate and low cobalamin levels in the serum, depending on the location of the SIBO and the number or species of bacteria involved.[72,76,78] Once exocrine pancreatic insufficiency is excluded, bacterial overgrowth is the most likely cause of low serum cobalamin.[76] Lack of protective IgA allows damage to enterocytes by bacteria, which leads to diarrhea.[71]

Because German shepherds are popular as pets and as working dogs where stools must be picked up for disposal, intermittent loose stools due to IgA deficiency[70–72] or IgA dysregulation[73,79] are unacceptable. Diminished intestinal mucosal production of IgA in German shepherds is probably due to defective synthesis or secretion of IgA rather than a lack of IgA-producing cells in the mucosa.[74] Likewise, the immune dysfunction that predisposes German shepherd dogs to deep pyoderma or anal furunculosis may be due to functionally defective T cells at the site of inflammation.[80,81]

Lymphocytic-plasmacytic enteritis may be a direct consequence of SIBO.[71,76] Enhanced permeability and histologic damage to jejunal mucosa was associated with confirmed SIBO in clinically normal beagles.[77] Antibiotic treatment to correct SIBO led to marked improvement in histologic lesions in a German shepherd.[76] Some investigators associate food allergy with low IgA levels.[64,67] The putative mechanism is that increased absorption of antigens is possible when IgA antibody is not present to bind to bacterial or food macromolecules before they penetrate mucosal barriers.[67,75] The antigens may stimulate IgG production within the lamina propria, explaining the presence of higher albumin and higher IgG in feces of German shepherds that were IgA deficient.[66]

Oxytetracycline and metronidazole, along with vitamin B12 supplementation, have been used to successfully treat SIBO in dogs.[72,76] If food allergy or damage to the intestinal mucosa from SIBO is suspected, a hypoallergenic food may be helpful in restoring and maintaining normal stool consistency.

SUMMARY

Inherited primary immunodeficiencies of dogs and cats may present as defects in neutrophil function, antibody production, complement activity, or cell-mediated immunity. Some deficiencies may be suspected because of lack of palpable lymph nodes on physical examination, history of persistent/recurrent infection, or changes in the hemogram. If immunodeficiencies are more readily considered in differential diagnoses, more will likely be recognized. Reference laboratories (Diagnostic Laboratory, College of Veterinary Medicine, Cornell University, Ithaca, NY 14853-6401, USA, www.vet.cornell.edu) offer additional tests to evaluate immune function.

As pet owners become more willing to pay for diagnostics because of the human-animal bond, primary care veterinarians will be better able to identify immunodeficient animals. Proper treatment or recommendations for referral earlier in a pet's life will enhance quality of life and quality of veterinary care.

REFERENCES

1. Abbas AK, Lichtman AH, Pober JS. Congenital and acquired immunodeficiencies. In: Cellular and molecular immunology. 4th edition. Philadelphia: W.B. Saunders Company; 2000. p. 445–67.
2. Tizard IR. Primary immunodeficiencies. In: Veterinary immunology, an introduction. 8th edition. St Louis (MO): Saunders Elsevier; 2009. p. 448–63.
3. Day MJ. Immunodeficiency disease in the dog. In: The 29th World Congress of the World Small Animal Veterinary Association Proceedings Online 2004. Rhodes (Greece). Available at: http://www.vin.com/proceedings/Proceedings. plx?CID5WSAVA2004&PID58598&Print51&O5Generic. Accessed February 14, 2010.
4. Bowles CA, Alsaker RD, Wolfle TL. Studies of the Pelger-Huët anomaly in Foxhounds. Am J Pathol 1979;96(1):237–47.
5. Tizard IR. Innate immunity: inflammation. In: Veterinary immunology, an introduction. 6th edition. Philadelphia: W.B. Saunders Company; 2000. p. 36–46.
6. Bauer TR Jr, Hai M, Tuschong LM, et al. Correction of the disease phenotype in canine leukocyte adhesion deficiency using ex vivo hematopoietic stem cell gene therapy. Blood 2006;108(10):3313–20.

7. Trowald-Wigh G, Ekman S, Hansson K, et al. Clinical, radiological and pathological features of 12 Irish setters with canine leucocyte adhesion deficiency. J Small Anim Pract 2000;41:211–7.

8. Debenham SL, Millington A, Kijas J, et al. Canine leucocyte adhesion deficiency in Irish red and white setters. J Small Anim Pract 2002;43:74–5.

9. Jobling AI, Ryan J, Augusteyn RC. The frequency of the canine leukocyte adhesion deficiency (CLAD) allele within the Irish setter population of Australia. Aust Vet J 2003;81(12):763–5.

10. Creevy KE, Bauer TR Jr, Tuschong LM, et al. Mixed chimeric hematopoietic stem cell transplant reverses the disease phenotype in canine leukocyte adhesion deficiency. Vet Immunol Immunopathol 2003;95:113–21.

11. Burkholder TH, Colenda L, Tuschong LM, et al. Reproductive capability in dogs with canine leukocyte adhesion deficiency treated with nonmyeloablative conditioning prior to allogeneic hematopoietic stem cell transplantation. Blood 2006; 108(5):1767–9.

12. Creel D, Collier LL, Leventhal AG, et al. Abnormal retinal projections in cats with the Chediak-Higashi syndrome. Invest Ophthalmol Vis Sci 1982;23(6): 798–801.

13. Collier LL, King EJ, Prieur DJ. Tapetal degeneration in cats with Chediak-Higashi syndrome. Curr Eye Res 1985;4(7):767–73.

14. Kramer JW, Davis WC, Prieur DJ. The Chediak-Higashi syndrome of cats. Lab Invest 1977;36(5):554–62.

15. Prieur DJ, Collier LL. Animal model of human disease: Chédiak-Higashi syndrome. Am J Pathol 1978;90(2):533–6.

16. Prieur DJ, Collier LL. Neutropenia in cats with the Chediak-Higashi syndrome. Can J Vet Res 1987;51:407–8.

17. Colgan SP, Gasper PW, Thrall MA, et al. Neutrophil function in normal and Chediak-Higashi syndrome cats following administration of recombinant canine granulocyte colony-stimulating factor. Exp Hematol 1992;20(10):1229–34.

18. Dale DC, Alling DW, Wolff SM. Cyclic hematopoiesis: the mechanism of cyclic neutropenia in grey collie dogs. J Clin Invest 1972;51:2197–204.

19. Chusid MJ, Bujak JS, Dale DC. Defective polymorphonuclear leukocyte metabolism and function in canine cyclic neutropenia. Blood 1975;46:921–30.

20. Dale DC, Graw RG Jr. Transplantation of allogeneic bone marrow in canine cyclic neutropenia. Science 1974;183:83–4.

21. Weiden PL, Robinett B, Graham TC, et al. Canine cyclic neutropenia, a stem cell defect. J Clin Invest 1974;53:950–3.

22. Allan FJ, Thompson KG, Jones BR, et al. Neutropenia with a probable hereditary basis in border collies. NZ Vet J 1996;44:67–72.

23. Shearman JR, Zhang QY, Wilton AN. Exclusion of CXCR4 as the cause of trapped neutrophil syndrome in Border Collies using five microsatellites on canine chromosome 19. Anim Genet 2006;37:72–89.

24. Shearman JR, Wilton AN. Elimination of neutrophil elastase and adaptor protein complex 3 subunit genes as the cause of trapped neutrophil syndrome (TNS) in border collies. Anim Genet 2007;38:188–9.

25. Wilton A. TNS DNA Border collie test results. Available at: http://www.bordercolliehealth.com/TNSdatabase.html. University of New South Wales, Australia. Accessed February 14, 2010.

26. Lanevschi A, Daminet S, Niemeyer GP, et al. Granulocyte colony-stimulating factor deficiency in a rottweiler with chronic idiopathic neutropenia. J Vet Intern Med 1999;13(1):72–5.

27. Renshaw HW, Davis WC. Canine granulocytopathy syndrome. Am J Pathol 1979; 95(3):731–44.
28. Couto CG, Krakowka S, Johnson G, et al. In vitro immunologic features of weimaraner dogs with neutropil abnormalities and recurrent infections. Vet Immunol Immunopathol 1989;23:103–12.
29. Hansen P, Clercx C, Henroteaux M, et al. Neutrophil phagocyte dysfunction in a weimaraner with recurrent infections. J Small Anim Pract 1995;36:128–31.
30. Studdert VP, Phillips WA, Studdert MJ, et al. Recurrent and persistent infections in related weimaraner dogs. Aust Vet J 1984;61(8):261–3.
31. Breitschwerdt EB, Brown TT, DeBuysscher EV, et al. Rhinitis, pneumonia and defective neutrophil function in the Doberman pinscher. Am J Vet Res 1987;48: 1054–62.
32. Meek K, Kienker L, Dallas C, et al. SCID in jack russell terriers: a new animal model of DNA-PKcs deficiency. J Immunol 2001;167:2142–50.
33. Felsburg PJ, Hartnett BJ, Henthorn PS, et al. Canine X-linked severe combined immunodeficiency. Vet Immunol Immunopathol 1999;69:127–35.
34. Somberg RL, Pullen RP, Casal ML, et al. A single nucleotide insertion in the canine interleukin-2 receptor gamma chain results in X-linked severe combined immunodeficiency disease. Vet Immunol Immunopathol 1995;47: 203–13.
35. Hartnett BJ, Henthorn PS, Moore PF, et al. Bone marrow transplantation for canine X-linked severe combined immunodeficiency. Vet Immunol Immunopathol 1999; 69:137–44.
36. Felsburg PJ, Somberg RL, Hartnett BJ, et al. Full immunologic reconstitution following nonconditioned bone marrow transplantation for canine X-linked severe combined immunodeficiency. Blood 1997;90(8):3214–21.
37. Goldschmidt MH, Kennedy JS, Kennedy DR, et al. Severe papillomavirus infection progressing to metastatic squamous cell carcinoma in bone marrow-transplanted X-linked SCID dogs. J Virol 2006;80(13):6621–8.
38. Day MJ. Possible immunodeficiency in related rottweiler dogs. J Small Anim Pract 1999;40:561–8.
39. Day MJ, Power C, Oleshko J, et al. Low serum immunoglobulin concentrations in related weimearaner dogs. J Small Anim Pract 1997;38:311–5.
40. Casal ML, Straumann U, Sigg C, et al. Congenital hypotrichosis with thymic aplasia in nine Birman kittens. J Am Anim Hosp Assoc 1994;30:600–2.
41. Wilkie BN, Markham RJF, Hazlett C. Deficient cutaneous response to PHA-P in healthy puppies from a kennel with a high prevalence of demodicosis. Can J Comp Med 1979;43:415–9.
42. McEwan NA. Mallassezia and Candida infections in bull terriers with lethal acrodermatitis. J Small Anim Pract 2001;42:291–7.
43. Jesyk PF, Haskins ME, MacKay-Smith WE, et al. Lethal acrodermatitis in bull terriers. J Am Vet Med Assoc 1986;188(8):833–9.
44. McEwan NA. Lethal acrodermatitis of bull terriers. Vet Rec 1990;127(4):95.
45. McEwan NA, McNeil PE, Thompson H, et al. Diagnostic features, confirmation and disease progression in 28 cases of lethal acrodermatitis of bull terriers. J Small Anim Pract 2000;41(11):501–7.
46. McEwan NA, Huang HP, Mellor DJ. Immunoglobulin levels in bull terriers suffering from lethal acrodermatitis. Vet Immunol Immunopathol 2003;96:235–8.
47. Roth JA, Kaeberle ML, Grier RL, et al. Improvement in clinical condition and thymus morphologic features associated with growth hormone treatment of immunodeficient dwarf dogs. Am J Vet Res 1984;45(6):1151–5.

48. Leisewitz AL, Spencer JA, Jacobson LS, et al. Suspected primary immunodeficiency syndrome in three related Irish wolfhounds. J Small Anim Pract 1997;38: 209–12.
49. Clercx C, Reichler I, Peeters D, et al. Rhinitis/bronchopneumonia syndrome in Irish Wolfhounds. J Vet Intern Med 2003;17:843–9.
50. Ameratunga R, Winkelstein JA, Brody L, et al. Molecular analysis of the third component of canine complement (C3) and identification of the mutation responsible for hereditary canine C3 deficiency. J Immunol 1998;160: 2824–30.
51. Tizard IR. The complement system. In: Veterinary immunology, an introduction. 6th edition. Philadelphia: W.B. Saunders Company; 2000. p. 170–9.
52. Lobetti R. Common variable immunodeficiency in miniature dachshunds affected with *Pneumonocystis carinii* pneumonia. J Vet Diagn Invest 2000;12: 39–45.
53. Lobetti RG, Leisewitz AL, Spencer JA. *Pneumocystis carinii* in the miniature dachshund: case report and literature review. J Small Anim Pract 1996;37: 280–5.
54. Lobetti RG. *Pneumocystis carinii* infection in miniature dachshunds. Comp Cont Educ Pract Vet 2001;23:320–4.
55. Meffert FJ. Pneumocystis pneumonia in two cavalier King Charles spaniel littermates. Aust Vet Pract 2009;39(1):2–9.
56. Sukura A, Saari S, Jarvinen AK, et al. *Pneumocysitis carinii* pneumonia in dogs— a diagnostic challenge. J Vet Diagn Invest 1996;8:124–30.
57. Watson PJ, Wotton P, Eastwood J, et al. Immunoglobulin deficiency in cavalier King Charles spaniels with *Pneumocystis* pneumonia. J Vet Intern Med 2006; 20:523–7.
58. Cabanes FJ, Roura X, Majo N, et al. *Pneumonocystis carinii* pneumonia in a Yorkshire terrier dog. Med Mycol 2000;38:451–3.
59. Furuta T, Nogami S, Kojima S, et al. Spontaneous *Pneumocystis carinii* infection in the dog with naturally acquired generalized demodicosis. Vet Rec 1994;134: 423–4.
60. Plechner AJ. IgM deficiency in 2 Doberman pinschers. Mod Vet Pract 1979;60:150.
61. Abeles V, Harrus S, Angles JM, et al. Hypertrophic osteodystrophy in six weimaraner puppies associated with systemic signs. Vet Rec 1999;145:130–4.
62. Harrus S, Waner T, Aizenberg I, et al. Development of hypertrophic osteodystrophy and antibody response in a litter of vaccinated weimaraner puppies. J Small Anim Pract 2002;43:27–31.
63. Foale RD, Herrtage ME, Day MJ. Retrospective study of 25 weimaraners with low serum immunoglobulin concentrations and inflammatory disease. Vet Rec 2003; 153:553–8.
64. Campbell KL, Neitzel C, Zuckermann FA. Immunoglobulin A deficiency in the dog. Canine Pract 1991;16(4):7–11.
65. Ginel PJ, Novales M, Lozano MD, et al. Local secretory IgA in dogs with low systemic IgA levels. Vet Rec 1993;132:321–3.
66. Littler RM, Batt RM, Lloyd DH. Total and relative deficiency of gut mucosal IgA in German shepherd dogs demonstrated by faecal analysis. Vet Rec 2006;158: 334–41.
67. Moroff SD, Hurvitz AI, Peterson ME, et al. IgA deficiency in shar pei dogs. Vet Immunol Immunopathol 1986;13:181–8.
68. Miller WH, Wellington JR, Scott DW. Dermatologic disorders of Chinese shar peis: 58 cases (1981–1989). J Am Vet Med Assoc 1992;200(7):986–90.

69. Glickman LT, Shofer FS, Payton AJ, et al. Survey of serum IgA, IgG, and IgM concentrations in a large beagle population in which IgA deficiency had been identified. Am J Vet Res 1988;49(8):1240–5.

70. Whitebread TJ, Batt RM, Garthwaite G. Relative deficiency of serum IgA in the German shepherd dog: a breed abnormality. Res Vet Sci 1984;37:350–2.

71. Batt RM, Barnes A, Rutgers HC, et al. Relative IgA deficiency and small intestinal bacterial overgrowth in German shepherd dogs. Res Vet Sci 1991;50:106–11.

72. Willard MD, Simpson RB, Fossum TW, et al. Characterization of naturally developing small intestinal bacterial overgrowth in 16 German shepherd dogs. J Am Vet Med Assoc 1994;204(8):1201–6.

73. Day MJ. Low IgA concentration in the tears of German shepherd dogs. Aust Vet J 1996;74(6):433–4.

74. German AJ, Hall EJ, Day MJ. Relative deficiency in IgA production by duodenal explants from German shepherd dogs with small intestinal disease. Vet Immunol Immunopathol 2000;76:25–43.

75. Norris CR, Gershwin LJ. Evaluation of systemic and secretory IgA concentrations and immunohistochemical stains for IgA-containing B cells in mucosal tissues of an Irish setter with selective IgA deficiency. J Am Anim Hosp Assoc 2003;39: 247–50.

76. Rutgers HC, Batt RM, Kelly DF. Lymphocytic-plasmacytic enteritis associated with bacterial overgrowth in a dog. J Am Vet Med Assoc 1988;192(12):1739–42.

77. Batt RM, Hall EJ, McLean L, et al. Small intestinal bacterial overgrowth and enhanced intestinal permeability in healthy beagles. Am J Vet Res 1992;53(10): 1935–40.

78. Batt RM, Needham JR, Carter MW. Bacterial overgrowth associated with a naturally occurring enteropathy in the German shepherd dog. Res Vet Sci 1983;35: 42–6.

79. Day MJ, Penhale WJ. Serum immunoglobulin A concentrations in normal and diseased dogs. Res Vet Sci 1988;45:360–3.

80. Day MJ. An immunopathological study of deep pyoderma in the dog. Res Vet Sci 1994;56:18–23.

81. Guilford WG. Primary immunodeficiency diseases of dogs and cats. Comp Cont Educ Pract Vet 1987;9(6):641–50.

Autoimmune Diseases in Small Animals

Laurel J. Gershwin, DVM, PhD

KEYWORDS

- Autoimmune disease • Canine • Feline
- Antinuclear antibodies • Systemic lupus erythematosus
- Autoimmune hemolytic anemia

The function of the immune system is to protect the host from pathogens. The complex system of humoral and cellular immune components that interact to provide this protection depends on an ability to differentiate self from nonself. Early in fetal development, the thymus "educates" fetal thymic lymphocytes so that those that enter the periphery and become mature T lymphocytes do not react in an adverse way with host cells and tissues and are able to assist in the elimination of pathogens and other foreign cells that enter the host. Nonetheless, there are situations in which an immune response may be generated such that self-tissues are attacked. These responses are referred to as autoimmune and, depending on which of the self-antigens the immune response is directed toward, clinical signs of disease occur and are relevant to the functions of those target tissues or organs. For example, in autoimmune hemolytic anemia, antibodies bind specifically with antigenic epitopes on self-erythrocytes causing loss of red blood cells and subsequent anemia.

Thymic education of fetal thymocytes takes place in the thymic cortex where there are epithelial cells that express a wide variety of tissue antigens and major histocompatibility (MHC) antigens class I and II. The immature T cells are "tested" for their ability to bind to self-MHC antigens. Those that do not bind at all are subject to induction of apoptosis and are eliminated. Those that bind too strongly are similarly disposed of. The T cells with ability to recognize MHC of self but do not bind strongly enough to elicit a cytotoxic event are retained. These cells become CD4 or CD8 T cells and can bind to MHC class II or MHC class I, respectively, whereas their T-cell receptor (TCR) for antigen has specificity for some foreign epitope. The TCRs are screened for reactivity to the promiscuously expressed tissue antigens on thymic epithelial cells, and those that react with any of these antigens are induced into apoptosis and eliminated from the T-cell pool that enters the periphery to seed the secondary lymphoid organs.

Department of Pathology, Microbiology & Immunology, School of Veterinary Medicine, One Shields Avenue, University of California, Davis, CA 95616, USA
E-mail address: ljgershwin@ucdavis.edu

Vet Clin Small Anim 40 (2010) 439–457
doi:10.1016/j.cvsm.2010.02.003
0195-5616/10/$ – see front matter © 2010 Elsevier Inc. All rights reserved.

vetsmall.theclinics.com

Although the majority of B cells are tolerized to self-antigens, the specificity of B-cell receptors on B lymphocytes is not as rigorously controlled as that of T lymphocytes. There are B cells present in the body that are capable of recognizing and binding to some self-epitopes. The lack of T cells reactive with those antigens, however, keeps the B cells in check because they require T-cell help to initiate an immune response and antibody production.

There are several well-recognized pathogenic mechanisms for induction of autoimmune responses, and there are also many autoimmune diseases for which there is no known reason for development of the autoimmune response. One well-recognized mechanism occurs when the target tissue is in a privileged site, such that the T and B cells were never exposed to its tissue specific antigens during development. These sites include central nervous system tissues, the lens of the eye, and sperm-forming cells in the male testicle. If a traumatic event exposes these tissues to the adult immune system, an immune attack on the organ or tissue is a common sequel. Another well-recognized mechanism occurs when there are shared antigenic epitopes between a host tissue and a pathogen, such as a virus or bacteria. The presence of helper T cells specific for the pathogen makes it possible for B cells that are not tolerized to the cross-reactive antigens to use those T cells to establish the costimulatory signals required for activation and differentiation into antibody-producing plasma cells. The resultant antibodies can then attack the self-tissues and evoke inflammation and tissue destruction. Such is the case in rheumatic fever and heart disease in human patients infected with group A streptococci that cross-react with myocardial antigens.

A less well understood mechanism for development of autoimmune responses is the loss of suppression, which in current immunologic terms involves an alteration in regulatory T cell function. In the 1980s, the concept of T suppressor cells that held autoreactive lymphocytes in check was expanded to explain development of autoimmune responses.

Recently, the discovery of T helper 17 (Th17) cells and their role in chronic inflammatory and autoimmune disorders has enhanced understanding of important regulatory mechanisms. Human patients with Hashimoto thyroiditis, a T cell–mediated autoimmune disease that dogs and human patients develop, showed increased levels of T cells synthesizing IL-17 and IL-22 in peripheral blood when compared with controls.[1] IL-17–secreting Th17 cells have been identified as active components in the pathogenesis of multiple sclerosis in human patients and immune-mediated experimental encephalitis in animal models.[2] II-17 is a proinflammatory cytokine and is implicated in the chronic autoimmune inflammation seen in rheumatoid arthritis (RA) patients.[3]

Autoimmune disease was first recognized as rheumatic disease in the 1800s and was later referred to by Ehrlich as horror autotoxicus. Since those early descriptions, myriad autoimmune diseases have been recognized in humans. The recognition of autoimmune disease in domestic animals has lagged somewhat behind that for humans. Currently, autoimmune etiology is implicated in a variety of inflammatory diseases in dogs and cats, with representative disorders affecting most body systems. Although the pathogenesis of these diseases vary, all are caused by antibody or T-cell responses to self-antigens.

SYSTEMIC AUTOIMMUNE DISEASE: SYSTEMIC LUPUS ERYTHEMATOSUS

Initially recognized in human patients, systemic lupus erythematosus (SLE) is the autoimmune disease with the most diverse clinical presentation. The cause of SLE is unknown, but it is characterized by the production of primarily nonorgan-specific autoantibodies. These autoantibodies are directed against self-molecules found in the cell nucleus. Autoantibodies to cell surface antigens are also found in this disease. In human patients there is a genetic predisposition for SLE (highest incidence is in African Americans) and a higher incidence rate in women.[4] Several MHC class II genes have been implicated.

In dogs there is also a genetic predisposition; it is most commonly seen in collies, German shepherds, and Shetland sheepdogs. Other breeds, such as Irish setters and poodles, may be affected. Several MHC class I antigens (DLA-A7) are associated with an increased incidence of SLE.[5] A canine patient presenting with SLE may show clinical signs relevant to the skin, kidney, joints, or hematologic system. The guidelines for diagnosis of SLE in human patients as established by the American College of Rheumatology include a positive antinuclear antibody (ANA) test or lupus erythematosus cell preparation and documented involvement of at least 2 body systems.[4] In a 1993 study, the most common clinical signs were polyarthritis (in 91% of cases), renal involvement (65%), and mucocutaneous disorders (60%). Only 13% of patients had hemolytic anemia. ANAs were detected using indirect immunofluorescence assay (IFA) at titers of 256 and over. These titers correlated with the severity and the stage of the disease.[6]

As discussed previously, diagnosis of SLE requires that patients have a positive ANA titer and the involvement of at least 2 body systems. In dogs with SLE, ANAs commonly recognize histones or soluble nuclear antigen whereas human ANA specificities favor double-stranded DNA as the antigen.[7] The ANA test is usually performed by IFA using fixed HEP-2 cells derived from mouse liver tissue as antigen. The pattern of immunofluorescence and the titer can be detected and reported. The speckled and homogeneous patterns are most commonly recognized in canine sera. A recent study examined 120 dogs with and without positive ANA and determined that in those showing involvement of 1 or more body systems suggestive of systemic autoimmune disease, a positive ANA test was most likely to be predictive for SLE whereas a positive ANA test in the absence of at least 1 body system involved was not a good predictor for diagnosis of SLE.[8] The presence of a decreased albumin/globulin ratio on blood analysis reflects the polyclonal activation of B cells with production of large amounts of immunoglobulin. Unlike the low albumin/globulin ratio in multiple myeloma, the densitometry tracing reveals a broad band reflecting the multiple clonality of the B cells that have been activated.

Pathogenic mechanisms in canine SLE involve development of immune complexes between antibodies specific for nuclear components and the liberated nuclear antigens in the circulation. When immune complexes deposit in kidney glomeruli, capillary networks in the joints, and the skin, a type III hypersensitivity reaction ensues and tissue damage results. Thus, fixation of complement liberates small fragments (C3a and C5a), which are chemotactic for neutrophils. The neutrophils release destructive enzymes in the tissues that contain immune complexes and inflammation and tissue necrosis occur. Resultant pathology gives rise to leaky glomerular capillaries and proteinuria, joint inflammation with resultant arthritis, and skin lesions. Some or all of these occur depending on the location of the immune reaction.

In SLE patients, other autoantibodies can occur, causing clinical signs relevant to different body systems. For example, if autoantibodies specific for erythrocyte antigens are made, hemolytic anemia may be part of the SLE complex. In this case, a Coombs test for antierythrocyte antibodies is positive and the hematologic system counts for 1 affected body system. Similarly the presence of antithrombocyte antibodies causes thrombocytopenia. The pathogenesis of both of these conditions involves a type II hypersensitivity reaction in which antibodies bind the target cells and opsonize for removal by the fixed phagocyte system in the spleen or complement-mediated lysis. Thus, it is understandable that SLE patients may present with a shifting leg lameness due to arthritis, kidney failure due to immune complex-mediated glomerularnephritis, or anemic crisis due to Coombs-positive anemia or bleeding from thrombocytopenia.

Immune-mediated polyarthritis is a common component of SLE. Arthrocentesis from hock and carpal joints reveals an increase in neutrophilic inflammation in the absence of microorganisms. Joint taps are useful to follow the response of a patient to immunosuppressive therapy.

SLE patients presenting with erythematous lesions on the face will likely have immune complex deposition at the dermal epidermal junction (**Fig. 1**). Lesions on the nasal planum are common. Immunofluorescence staining of a biopsy from affected areas when stained with antisera specific for IgG or third component of complement (C3) shows a fluorescent band at the dermal epidermal junction. This lupus band is characteristic for SLE skin lesions (see **Fig. 1**B). There is a similar skin pathology that occurs in the absence of other body system involvement and in which patient serum is negative for ANAs; this condition is referred to as discoid lupus (DL). The lesions on the nasal planum are similar. DL and the skin manifestation of SLE are exacerbated by direct exposure to UV light.

Although the pathogenesis of SLE is well understood, the inciting cause for induction of the autoimmune response is usually elusive. Virus infection or exposure to environmental toxicants and other chemicals is often proposed. There are some definitive links to causal agents in the case of feline hyperthyroid patients treated with 6- propylthiouracil. These patients develop a lupus-like syndrome with formation of antibodies to native DNA. The development of this syndrome seems to be dose dependent.[9]

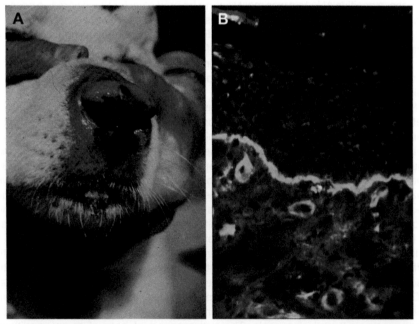

Fig. 1. (*A*) Erosive lesions on nasal planum in canine SLE. (*B*) Direct immunofluorescence on biopsy (from lesions in [*A*]) using antisera against canine IgG shows antibody binding at dermal epidermal junction, the lupus band.

ORGAN SYSTEM–SPECIFIC AUTOIMMUNE DISEASE

Pathogenic mechanisms for organ-specific autoimmune diseases most commonly involve the development of autoantibodies specific for 1 or more antigens on the target tissue. The destruction of the targeted cells occurs by a type II hypersensitivity mechanism in which antibodies bind the cells and cause lysis/membrane damage leading to cell death or removal by the fixed macrophages in liver and splenic sinusoids. In some instances, the autoimmune effector is sensitized T lymphocytes. In this case, the target organ is infiltrated with lymphocytes and other mononuclear cells. When T cells mediate damage, destruction of cells and tissue occurs by cell-mediated induction of apoptosis.

AUTOIMMUNE DISEASES OF THE HEMATOLOGIC SYSTEM
Immune-Mediated Hemolytic Anemia

In dogs, immune-mediated hemolytic anemia (IMHA) is a common cause of anemia, and in cats it is somewhat less common but not infrequent. Canine patients are often middle-aged female dogs, but in cats, males, at least in 1 study, were overrepresented.[10] On presentation, IMHA patients show depression, pallor, and sometimes jaundice. The diagnosis of IMHA is suspected when a hemogram reveals spherocytosis and a regenerative anemia; this is usually accompanied by a positive Coombs test. IMHA can be idiopathic or instigated by 1 of several drugs, such as β-lactam antibiotics.[11] In the latter case, metabolic products of the drug bind to erythrocytes creating a new epitope, which stimulates the production of antibodies that bind to the erythrocyte, fix complement, and initiate cell lysis or removal by fixed phagocytes in the spleen. It is likely, but not yet well documented, that overvaccination may serve as an inciting cause of IMHA in dogs. Polyclonal activation of B cells could induce autoantibody formation, particularly in genetically predisposed dogs.

A positive result from the direct Coombs test is a useful predictor of disease in dogs, but in cats, false-positive results are more frequent than in dogs. One study of IMHA in cats showed that the median packed cell volume on presentation was 12%. In more than 50% of the cats, the anemia was not regenerative. Additional abnormal laboratory results included leukocytosis, lymphocytosis, hyperbilirubinemia, and hyperglobulimemia.[12]

The pathogenesis of IMHA varies depending on the isotype and specificity of the autoantibody produced. In IMHA, erythrocytes are targeted by antierythrocyte antibodies and anemia is the dominant clinical sign. When hemoglobinuria and hemaglobinemia are present, IgM is usually the predominant antibody because it causes complement-mediated lysis with subsequent icterus and hemoglobinemia. In contrast, an IgG antibody (so-called incomplete antibody) leads to anemia with low hematocrit and no hemolysis. This latter type of presentation is caused primarily by loss of erythrocytes from phagocytic destruction after being opsonized by IgG antibody. These cases generally show splenomegaly and sometimes also hepatomegaly.[10] Immune-mediated anemia in which the erythrocytes are agglutinated at cold temperatures by cold agglutinins has been characterized.[10]

There are some dog breeds that have an increased incidence of IMHA. These include cocker spaniel, miniature schnauzer, beagle, Samoyed, and old English sheepdog.[13] An association between a DLA class II haplotype and an increased incidence of IMHA has been described.[14] In a study of 108 patients with Coombs-positive anemia, the 2 haplotypes that were increased relative to a breed-matched control cohort were: DLA-DRB1*00601/DQA1*005011/DQB1*00701, reported in dogs with warm reactive agglutinins; and DLA-DRB1*015/DQA1*00601/DQB1*00301 in dogs with both warm and cold reactive agglutinins. These results are similar to the associations found for human IMHA patients.

Treatment of IMTP, as of other diseases of autoimmune origin, requires vigorous immunosuppressive therapy, usually immunosuppressive doses of corticosteroids. Adjunct therapy may include the use of intravenous human immunoglobulin (to block Fc receptors on phagocytes), transfusion (only for animals in dire need of red blood cells), and other supportive care for animals in anemic crisis.[11,15]

IMHA can occur by itself or with immune-mediated thrombocytopenia (IMTP), a condition known as Evans syndrome. The combination of erythrocyte loss and thrombocyte depletion creates a severe disease in which erythrocyte loss by immune depletion is supplemented by loss due to bleeding. In 1 study of 21 cases of IMHA and IMTP, there was overrepresentation of Airedale terriers and Dobermans. Less than 50% of the dogs survived for 30 days after original hospitalization, usually for bleeding disorders.[16]

Immune-Mediated Thrombocytopenia

Primary idiopathic IMTP occurs without a known inciting cause and is more common in middle-aged female dogs. Cocker spaniels and old English sheepdogs are overrepresented. Patients with IMTP may present with prolonged bleeding, petechia, or ecchymosis. The presence of antibodies reactive with thrombocytes can be confirmed using the antimegakaryocyte antibody test on bone marrow or an indirect immunofluorescent evaluation of platelet-bound antibodies (PBAs) in the peripheral blood using flow cytometry. The detection of these antibodies is diagnostic for IMTP. In 1 recent study involving 83 thrombocytopenic dogs, 45% were found to have PBAs, as determined by flow cytometry.[17] Increased megakaryopoiesis was observed in all dogs that were suspected of having ITP but in only 39% of dogs without PBAs.

Treatment of IMTP involves the use of immunosuppressive therapy (usually prednisone and cyclophosphamide to induce remission and azathioprine to maintain remission). The use of blood or packed cell transfusion depends on the hematocrit and need for blood. In a recent study, Horgan and colleagues[18] found that splenectomy as an adjunct to immunosuppressive therapy was associated with improved outcome. Response to immunosuppressive therapy usually results in an increase of platelet levels to normal. Treatment of IMTP with intravenous human immunoglobulin has been evaluated by several groups. This procedure is often used in human patients with IMTP, as in IMHA, and is based on the principle that the human immunoblobulin blocks the Fc receptors on mononuclear cells in patients, thus precluding removal of opsonized platelets. In 1 small study, the use of this treatment seemed to result in rapid rise of platelet counts and was not associated with adverse side effects.[19]

Idiopathic IMTP is most common; however, IMTP can occur secondary to drug therapy or infection. Several reported cases of ITP were linked to consumption of medications (anticonvulsants or antibiotics)—these cases are secondary ITP. In 1 study, 44 dogs infected naturally with *Leishmania infantum* were divided into those with and those without thrombocytopenia. Blood was tested for PBAs by IFA and 19 of 20 dogs with thrombocytopenia and 13 of 24 dogs without thrombocytopenia were positive by IFA. In contrast, 0 of 10 uninfected normal dogs were positive for PBAs.[20]

Immune-Mediated Neutropenia

Loss of neutrophils by immune destruction is the least common of the immune-mediated hematologic diseases. The presence of antibodies reactive with neutrophils has been documented, however, in several human syndromes and in dogs. Neutropenia can occur alone or in conjunction with thrombocytopenia. In 1 case report, immune-mediated neutropenia and thrombocytopenia was described in 3 giant schnauzer dogs.[21]

Two of these dogs had antineutrophil antibodies that were demonstrated by indirect agglutination (using Coombs reagent); in the third, IFA was used and it failed to detect antineutrophil antibodies. Patients with neutropenia present may present with recurrent bacterial infections due to the loss of a primary innate defense mechanism.

AUTOIMMUNE DISEASES OF THE ENDOCRINE SYSTEM
Autoimmune Thyroiditis

Autoimmune thyroiditis (AT), Hashimoto disease, is one of the most common autoimmune diseases in humans. It is characterized by infiltration of the thyroid gland with lymphocytes. Loss of thyroid function results in hypothyroidism. Development of antithyroxin antibodies is seen in 60% to 80% of these patients; in addition, antibodies to thyroperoxidase are present in up to 95% of patients and are considered to be superior as a predictive indicator of disease.[22]

Hypothyroidism is a common disorder of dogs, with certain breeds showing enhanced predisposition. Primary hypothyroidism in which the thyroid is infiltrated by lymphocytes is considered an immune-mediated disease, with histologic similarities to Hashimoto thyroiditis in humans. Antibodies to circulating T3 or to T4 are often detectable. The development of clinical signs of lethargy, dermatologic changes, and obesity are not usually seen until at least 75% of the gland has been destroyed. Measurement of blood levels of T4 is below normal, and up to 80% of these patients have detectable autoantibodies to thyroglobulin.[23] In dogs, hypothyroidism is most often manifested in middle age and is associated with obesity, mental dullness, alopecia primarily on the trunk, often secondary pruritic seborrhea sicca with or without otitis externa, hyperpigmentation, myxedema, and weakness. Other body systems can also be affected including the cardiovascular, gastrointestinal, and hematologic systems. Anemia is commonly associated with untreated AT.

There are many purebred dog breeds that have a higher than normal incidence of AT. Some of these include Doberman pinschers, golden retrievers, beagles, old English sheepdogs, Rhodesian ridgebacks, and many others. The disease is far less common in mixed breed dogs. Recent studies on MHC polymorphisms in affected dogs have identified several DLA antigens with increased representation in AT-affected dogs. Kennedy and colleagues[24] have identified a significant association between DLA-DQA1*00101 with hypothyroidism. These investigators note that several breeds (Siberian husky, shih tzu, and Yorkshire terrier) that are not associated with AT have a low frequency of expression of DLA-DQA1*00101. Immunoendocrinopathy syndromes may occur in AT dogs, with patients developing first AT and then type 1 diabetes mellitus (DM) or hypoadrenocorticism.[23] This is not surprising because there is evidence that the DLA-DQA1*001 allele is associated with DM and AT.[25] In a recent study using giant schnauzers and Hovawart dogs, Ferm and colleagues examined birth cohorts for the presence of antithyroid autoantibodies (ATAs) and for elevated thyrotropin levels. Although both breeds had members with clinical hypothyroidism present, the number of dogs testing positive for ATAs and having high thyrotropin levels was greater than the number of dogs with clinical disease, indicating the potential prognostic value of ANA and thyrotropin level testing in breeds predisposed to AT.[26]

Detection of ATAs in serum of hypothyroid dogs is a useful diagnostic aid. The role of these antibodies in pathogenesis, however, is not established. Studies performed by Choi and colleagues[27] have demonstrated that there is a Th1 skew in AT patients. The destructive role of the lymphocytes infiltrating the gland is likely the predominant pathogenic mechanism, whereas the antibodies are considered by some to be a result of tissue damage.

Treatment of dogs with AT involves supplementation with sodium levothyroxine daily at a dosage that ultimately brings the T4 level within the normal range. Most dogs respond well to thyroid supplementation. Immunosuppressive therapy is not usually used, because by the time patients are diagnosed, the damage to the gland has been done.

Autoimmune Diabetes Mellitus

DM is common in dogs and has an onset usually between 4 and 14 years of age. Female dogs are affected more frequently than male dogs. There is a breed predisposition, suggesting an underlying genetic component. A typical presentation involves polydypsia, polyuria, polyphagia, and weight loss. These signs are comparable with those of human DM patients. Cataract formation is common. Hypoinsulinemia prevents the use of blood glucose by cells and a resultant hyperglucosemia and glucosuria results. Ketosis is a potential complication of untreated DM.[28]

The pathogenesis of insulin-dependent DM in dogs does not always involve autoimmune destruction of the pancreatic beta cells. Other causes include pancreatitis, infection, and insulin antagonistic diseases. Canine DM most closely resembles DM in humans. The presence of circulating antibodies to insulin and to beta cell antigens has been documented, but the role of autoimmunity in beta cell loss is still under study. One study showed a 50% incidence of antibodies to islet cells in newly diagnosed cases of DM.[29] In human patients, autoantibodies to GAD65 (a 65-kDA form of glutamic acid decarboxylase) and to protein tyrosine phosphatase receptor (IA-2 antigen) have been demonstrated. These are 2 important antigens expressed by beta cells of the pancreas.[30] Davison and colleagues[31] studied 30 dogs with DM for serologic evidence of autoreactivity to GAD65 or the IA-2 antigen. Using cloned and expressed canine versions of these antigens, they found that 2 of the 30 diabetic dogs had significant reactivity to both antigens, and 2 other dogs reacted significantly to GAD65 and 1 dog reacted to IA-2 but not GAD65. As in the case of antibodies to thyroid antigens, a role in pathogenesis has not been demonstrated.

The breed predisposition for DM prompted a study by Catchpole and colleagues[25] on the potential association with MHC genes. Using 530 diabetic dogs and 1000 controls, this group examined DLA associations and found 3 haplotypes associated with DM in dogs. These were DLA-DRB1*009=DQA1*001=DQB1*008. These haplotypes were also common in the diabetes-prone breeds (Samoyed, cairn terrier, and Tibetan terrier) and rare in several breeds in which DM is not common.

AUTOIMMUNE SKIN DISEASE
Discoid Lupus

More than half of canine patients with SLE have involvement of the skin. The skin lesions are often on the face. The term *lupus*, Greek for wolf, was originally coined because the facial rash on human patients (butterfly-shaped area of erythema over the bridge of the nose and under the eyes) gave the patient's face a wolf-like appearance. The lupus rash is also exacerbated by sunlight. Canine SLE patients may have alopecia and erythema in a similar location (see **Fig. 1**A). DL is an autoimmune disease in which the lesions are similar to those of lupus but in the absence of a positive ANA and without involvement of other body systems. Biopsy of a lupus skin lesion stained for immunofluorescence using anti-IgG or anti-C3 reveals the presence of a band of fluorescence along the dermal-epidermal junction. This lupus band is diagnostic for DL (see **Fig. 1**B).

When the lesions characteristic of lupus are seen without a positive ANA test and in the absence of involvement of other body systems, the disease is called DL. Lesions are located on the nasal planum but can also occur on ear pinnae and around eyes. The disease is seen not uncommonly in dogs but is rare in cats. The prognosis is more favorable for this form of the disease. Treatment with corticosteroids and protection of the nasal planum from UV radiation by using topical sunscreen is indicated. Often topical glucocorticoids or cyclosporine ointment are sufficient for treatment, but in more severe cases systemic corticosteroids may be needed.[32]

Bullous Skin Diseases

Among the autoimmune skin diseases, the pemphigus complex of skin disease is one of the most commonly seen. This disease complex is characterized by the formation of vesicles in the skin; the subsequent rupture of these vesicles creates erosions that leave areas of the skin vulnerable to infection. The underlying pathology is instigated by the formation of antibodies against the cellular adhesion molecule, desmoglein 3. Binding of these antibodies causes the epithelial cells to detach from each other, creating acantholysis. There are several distinct diseases within this complex, some more severe than others. The difference in pathology is based on which epithelial layers are affected by the immune reaction.

The least severe form of the pemphigus diseases is pemphigus erythematosus. This disease affects mainly dogs and is most common in German shepherds, collies, and Shetland sheepdogs. It is uncommon in cats. The lesions are superficial and limited to the nose and around the eyes and ears. The oral cavity is not involved and the lesions are only mildly pruritic.

Pemphigus foliaceus is characterized by acantholysis in the most superficial layers of the epidermis. It is the most common of these diseases and is seen in both dogs and cats. The disease is seen in all breeds and both genders and shows no age predisposition. An increased incidence has been reported in the chow chow and the Akita breeds, however. Lesions are often first seen on the bridge of the nose and around the eyes. The ear pinnae are also affected and the footpads may show hyperkeratosis. In dogs, mucosal involvement does not usually occur. In cats, however, lesions may be seen around the nail beds and around the nipples.[33]

Pemphigus vulgaris is by far the most severe form of the pemphigus complex; fortunately, it is also the rarest form. The autoantibodies are directed to antigens on cells that are near the dermal-epidermal junction. Thus the binding of the autoantibodies and subsequent loss of cellular adhesion triggers acantholysis deep within the epidermis. Lesions consisting of bullae, erosions, and ulcers occur on mucosal surfaces (oral cavity, anus, conjunctiva, and so forth), at mucocutaneous junctions, and on the trunk, particularly in areas of skin-to-skin contact, such as axilla and groin. Systemic signs of illness, including fever, depression, and anorexia, are common.[34]

Diagnosis of the pemphigus diseases involves using dermatohistology and immunofluorescence or immunohistochemistry on biopsy specimens to demonstrate the deposition of antibody at the intercellular sites (**Fig. 2**). The presence of honeycomb-type fluorescence after staining with anti-IgG fluorescein is characteristic of the pemphigus complex.

On dermatohistology, pathologists recognize the presence of superbasilar clefts and vesicles in pemphigus vulgaris; in pemphigus foliaceus, the appearance of subcorneal pustules containing neutrophils and acantholytic cells is characteristic.[32–35]

Treatment of these diseases involves systemic immunosuppressive therapy and antibiotic treatment as needed when secondary infection is present. In permphigus erythematosus, the mildest form of the disease, often topical glucocorticoid therapy or cyclosporine topical treatment suffices. For the most severe form, high doses of corticosteroids are often supplemented with other immunosuppressive drugs, such

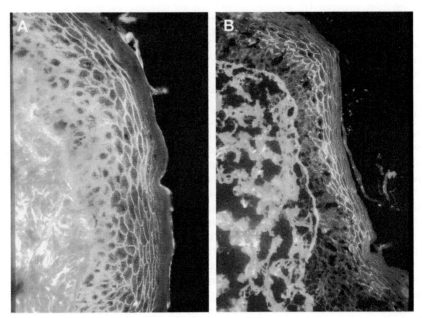

Fig. 2. Direct immunofluorescence on skin biopsy from a dog with pemphigus vulgaris. Section was stained with anti-canine IgG-FITC. Intercellular staining indicates the binding of autoantibodies to desmoglein 3 (*A, B*).

as azothoiprine (dogs only). The prognosis for the milder forms, pemphigus erythematosus, is good, but for pemphigus vulgaris the prognosis is at best fair and often poor. Lifetime immunosuppressive therapy is often required.

Bullous pemphigoid is a rare autoimmune skin disease in which the autoantibodies are directed against the lamina lucida (the basement membrane). Resultant lesions are the result of separation of the epidermis from the dermis. Very fragile vesicles result, which are not usually visualized in tact but rapidly become deep ulcers. Areas commonly affected include the head and neck, ear pinnae, ventral abdomen, and mucocutaneous junctions. The disease has been reported in dogs and cats.[35]

The nature and role of autoantibodies in the pemphigus diseases has been studied in dogs. In 1 study, 82% of dogs (n = 64) with pemphigus foliaceus had circulating IgG4 antibodies to keratinocytes as demonstrated by IFA on neonatal mouse skin. Serum from normal dogs frequently contained antikeratinocyte antibodies of the IgG4 subclass. Only those sera with IgG4 antibodies were associated with production of characteristic lesions in mouse skin after passive serum transfer. Thus the investigators concluded that IgG4 may be the pathogenic antibody as in the case of human pemphigus.[36] An earlier study had shown that circulating anti–desmoglein 3 IgG antibodies capable of dissociating keratinocytes are present in dogs with PV.[37] In 1 case study, the potential usefulness of serial IFA titers for antidesmoglein antibodies to demonstrate the effectiveness of therapy was illustrated. A progressive drop in antibody titers was associated with clinical improvement.[38]

AUTOIMMUNE DISEASES OF THE MUSCULOSKELETAL SYSTEM
Myasthenia Gravis

Myasthenia gravis (MG) is a disease that causes abnormal weakness and fatigue. It is seen in humans, dogs, cats, and ferrets.[39,40] In dogs, there is a congenital syndrome with this name, but the acquired form has an autoimmune pathogenesis. The underlying problem for both forms is a lack of postsynaptic nicotinic acetylcholine receptors; in the congenital form, the deficiency is due to a genetic mutation, whereas in the acquired form, the loss of acetylcholine receptors is a result of autoimmune attack. Formation of autoantibodies against these receptors triggers receptor degradation. The antibodies also block receptors so that acetylcholine released in the neuromuscular junction cannot bind to its receptor. Ultimately, the IgG antibodies fix complement (type II hypersensitivity) and cause receptor destruction. Thus, the nerve impulse carried to the muscle by acetylcholine does not transmit and the muscle is unable to contract. The degree of receptor destruction affects the severity of the weakness. An affected dog may present with muscle weakness of the skeletal system, but difficulty in swallowing and ultimately in breathing occurs when the disease progresses to involve muscles of mastication and respiratory skeletal muscle. Facial paralysis and megaesophagus are common and many dogs present with only these focal signs.

There seems to be a genetic predisposition for this disease in dogs and cats, although the disease is seen in many breeds. A retrospective study of more than 1000 cases showed that breeds with the highest risk of MG were Akita, terriers (except for Jack Russell), German shorthaired pointers, and Chihuahuas.[41] A similar survey of feline cases revealed that the there is a breed predisposition for acquired MG in Abyssinians (and related Somalis). There is a reported association with malignancy of the thymus in some cases.[42,43] In cats, acquired MG is sometimes associated with the presence of a cranial mediastinal mass.[44,45]

Diagnosis can be enhanced by observing the response to treatment with anticholinesterase drugs (such as edrophonium chloride), because these drugs allow the acetylcholine to remain longer in the synapse facilitating binding to those receptors that remain intact. Long-term use of these drugs is also suggested for patient management.

Testing for the presence of serum antibodies specific for the postsynaptic nicotinic acetylcholine receptors provides confirmation of the diagnosis for this disease. Upright feeding is recommended for dogs with megaesophagus. Surgical removal of thymomas, if present, is often performed. As in other autoimmune diseases, the use of immunosuppressive drugs can prevent further deterioration by halting the further destruction of acetylcholine receptors.[46]

A recent study has determined the nature of the antigenic epitope targeted by anti-acetylcholine receptor antibodies in human MG. The main immunogenic region is a conformation-dependent epitope on the extracellular apex of alpha-1 subunit of the muscle nicotinic acetylcholine receptor. This epitope was reported to be recognized by human, canine, and feline antiacetylcholine receptor antibodies.[47]

Rheumatoid Arthritis

Since the late 1970s, a syndrome in dogs similar to RA of humans has been recognized. In a signature case, a miniature poodle presented with chronic hind limb lameness. The presence of a polyclonal gammopathy, elevated leukocyte counts in the absence of infection in joint fluid, radiographic evidence of joint space narrowing in the carpal joints, and areas of subchondral lucency were compatible with the diagnosis of RA. In addition, a test for rheumatoid factor was positive. The dog was treated with prednisone with good response to long-term therapy.[48] This presentation is classic for the disease. The presence of joint stiffness, often first thing in the morning or after inactivity, is often accompanied with depression and anorexia. There is symmetric swelling of affected joints. RA must be differentiated from polyarthritis associated with SLE; animals with the former condition are negative for ANA whereas the latter are positive. Radiographic findings in RA generally show far more joint destruction with subchondral bone loss, whereas joints affected in polyarthritis of SLE lack these destructive lesions.

It has been recognized for some time that proinflammatory cytokines are important in pathogenesis of the disease.[49] Recently, the role of tumor necrosis factor α (TNF-α), interleukin 6 (IL)-6, and IL-1 in synovial fluid in pathogenesis of RA has formed the basis for new therapies based on blocking the effects of these cytokines. Clinical trials using antagonists of IL-1, TNF-α, and IL-6 receptor blockers have shown encouraging results in human patients.[50,51] One study on canine RA patients showed a 30-fold increase of matrix metalloprotease-3 over its inhibitor, tissue inhibitor of matrix metalloprotease-3, in RA dogs when compared with dogs with ruptured anterior cruciate ligament. This pattern correlated with levels of IL-1, IL-12, and transforming growth factor β. It is likely that Th17 cells play a role in initiation of the proinflammatory cytokine production. The presence of these cytokines in the joint fluid stimulates cartilage degradation by the metalloproteases. Thus, the lesion is lytic and accompanied by a synovial inflammation with lymphocyte and neutrophil accumulation, resulting in a fibrous vascular network, called pannus.[52]

The diagnosis of RA includes finding evidence of autoantibodies in serum or synovial fluid. The classic RA factor is an autoantibody directed against a self-immunoglobulin; IgG is most common (for assay details, see later discussion). Other autoantibodies may be directed to type II collagen and glycosaminoglycans. These autoantibodies are thought to have a role in joint destruction.

As with other autoimmune diseases, there are genetic predispositions for RA. In humans, there is an association of HLA-DRB1 with RA. Ollier and colleagues[53] sought to examine canine RA patients to see if a similar predisposition occurs in dogs. They found that several DLA alleles were associated with an increased risk of RA. These are DLA-DRB1*002, DRB1*009, and DRB1*018.

The nature of the initiating cause of RA is not clear in humans or in dogs. There is an association, however, with several infectious disease agents in both species. In the dog, immune complexes consisting of canine distemper virus and anticanine distemper virus antibodies were present in joint fluid of RA patients.[54,55] *Borrelia burgdorferi* has also been implicated in RA in 2 dogs recovering from *Borrelia* infection that were rheumatoid factor positive and progressed to RA.[56]

The prognosis for RA in humans and dogs is not good, particularly if the disease has progressed to joint destruction when therapy is instituted. Current anticytokine therapies show promise in human patients with RA. These include infliximab (a monoclonal antibody to TNF-α) and etanercept (a recombinant TNF-α receptor). Clinical trials with these new immunomodulatory preparations in dogs have yet to be published. In dogs, nonsteroidal anti-inflammatory drugs are often used initially, with corticosteroids, and more aggressive immunosuppressive therapy with methotrexate and gold salts is reserved for the most severe cases.

AUTOIMMUNE DISEASES OF THE EYE
Canine Uveodermatologic Syndrome (Vogt-Koyanagi-Harada Syndrome)

Vogt-Koyanagi-Harada syndrome (VKH) in humans is associated with an autoimmune attack on melanin containing cells. In dogs, the production of autoantibodies against uveal melanocytes results in granulomatous panuveitis and loss of skin and hair pigmentation. The condition is rare in dogs but is seen most frequently in the Akita breed. A recent study of canine VKH showed an association with increased frequency of DQA1*00201 in the Akita breed.[57] Other affected breeds include the Samoyed, chow chow, Siberian husky, Irish setter, old English sheepdog, and several other breeds.

The presenting signs of VKH are usually ocular, with acute onset of anterior uveitis, keratic precipitates, hyphema, and diminished pupillary reflex. Dermatologic signs may occur concurrently or slightly later than those affecting the eye. A well-demarcated symmetric depigmentation of the nose, lips, and eyelids is characteristic. Treatment of VKH involves vigorous ocular therapy to prevent blindness. The use of topical glucocorticoids and 1% atropine in the eye is accompanied with systemic immunosuppressive therapy with oral prednisone or methylprednisolone. If there is no or little response, then cyclosporine and oral azathioprine or cyclophosphamide can be used. Lifetime therapy is usually required.[58]

Investigators attempted to reproduce the lesions of VKH experimentally by immunizing Akita dogs with peptides derived from tyrosinase-related protein 1. The resulting autoimmune disease was similar to the spontaneous disease in Akitas.[59] This type of study may lead to better definition of the autoantigens important in VKH in humans and dogs.

LABORATORY METHODS FOR DETECTION OF AUTOIMMUNE DISEASE
Antinuclear Antibody Testing

ANAs are antibodies with specificity for nucleic acids and nucleoproteins. They are found in serum of people and animals. Although these antibodies are not normal, low levels are sometimes found in older patients or transiently in patients post trauma. Some infections can induce development of a positive ANA. High serum levels (titers >100), however, are associated with autoimmune diseases. Detection of ANAs in serum is an important parameter for making a diagnosis of SLE.

The most common method for detection of ANAs is an IFA. Green fluorescence of nuclei from a human hepatoma cell line (HEP-2 cells) is present after fixation to permeabilize the cells and subsequent incubation with serum from the patient. Patient serum antibodies are identified after further incubation with a fluorescein-tagged reagent that detects dog IgG. It is customary to initially test sera at a 1:20 dilution. If positive results are seen, then serial dilutions are tested to determine a titer. The titer is determined by looking for the last dilution of serum that gives a positive nuclear fluorescence comparable to the positive control serum.

In addition to a titer, the positive ANA test provides a description of the pattern of fluorescence. The speckled and homogeneous patterns are seen in cases of canine SLE and related syndromes.[60] Other patterns include nucleolar and rim staining, which are less commonly seen.

Detection of ANA is sensitive but not a specific test for autoimmune disease. In 1 study on *Leishmania infantum*, antihistone antibodies were found in 39% of dogs without glomerulonephritis and 88% with glomerulonephritis. In this study, there was a positive correlation between serum creatinine levels and antihistone titers.[61] Other studies have demonstrated high titers of ANA in dogs infected with vector-borne agents: *Ehrlichia canis*, 17% of seroreactors, and *Bartonella vinsonii* (berkhoffii), 75% of seroreactors.[62] In addition, treatment with certain drugs can induce development of ANA in some patients. Implicated drugs include griseofulvin, penicillin, sulfonamides, tetracyclines, phenytoin, and procainamide.

Detection of ANA by other assay methods is reported in the literature. The IFA using *Crithidia luciae,* if positive, indicates that antibodies to double-stranded DNA are present, because the kinetoplast of these protozoa contains only double-stranded DNA. In humans this is the best assay for ANAs in SLE.[63] Other antigens in the nucleus can be detected using enzyme-linked immunosorbent assay (ELISA) or immunoblot. In

1 study, the presence of antibodies to the Sm nuclear antigen and ribonuclear protein was demonstrated.[64] Double immunodiffusion testing to demonstrate precipitating antibodies specific for nuclear antigens has been applied to canine serum samples. In 1 study, the presence of precipitating antibodies to ribonuclear protein and Sm antigen was associated with the speckled pattern of immunofluorescence.[65] A recent follow-up study used a line blot assay (Inno-Lia ANA), commonly used in human diagnostics, to evaluate nuclear antigen specificities in ANA-positive dog sera. Antibodies to small nuclear ribonuclear protein antigens were detected in 6 of 20 ANA-positive canine sera, and 2 of the samples reacted with SMB antigen.[66] Thus it seems that some of the newly developed diagnostic test kits used in human diagnostic laboratories will be applicable to canine patients. There is less information available on the specificity of ANA in cats.

The usefulness of the ANA test in dogs with SLE has been demonstrated in clinical cases diagnosed of high (eg, 1:3200) titers that have been followed over time during treatment with immunosuppressive drugs. It is not uncommon to see the titer fall to negative or near negative (1:40) after chronic treatment.

DETECTION OF ORGAN-SPECIFIC AUTOANTIBODIES

Diagnosis of organ-specific autoimmune disease involves the detection of cell specific autoantibodies. For some diseases, such as IMHA, this is a common procedure, with the Coombs test serving as a gold standard. The Coombs test is the primary diagnostic test for IMHA. A recent study by Warman and colleagues[67] compared the value of using a polyvalent versus a monovalent Coombs reagent. They found that when erythrocytes were screened with anti-IgG, anti-IgM, and anti-C3 separately at both 4°C and 37°C, the test became significantly more sensitive than screening at 37°C with polyvalent Coombs reagent.

For other diseases, such as DM, the detection of antibodies binding to pancreatic islet cells is not a common procedure. Some of the more specific tests are not performed in all veterinary diagnostic laboratories but require that samples be sent to specialists in the area. For example, the assay for the detection of autoantibodies to the postsynaptic acetylcholine receptors in cases of MG is performed primarily at University of California, San Diego (laboratory of Dr G.D. Shelton). In general, the most common method for detection of tissue-specific antibodies is IFA or immunoperoxidase using patient sera on normal homologous tissue. Direct immunofluorescence or immunoperoxidase staining is often used on biopsy samples from tissues with suspected immunoglobulin binding or complex deposition. Hence, in skin from SLE- or DL-affected dogs, the incubation of a biopsy from patients with fluorescein isothiocyanate or enzyme-labeled antisera specific for canine IgG can reveal the presence of bound antibody at the dermal-epidermal junction. Kidney biopsy samples from SLE patients with kidney involvement when stained with similar reagents reveal the deposition of immune complexes. The use of antisera specific for the C3 can also be used to detect immune complex deposition.

THERAPEUTIC APPROACHES TO AUTOIMMUNE DISEASE

Autoimmune disease is caused by an uncontrolled immune response against self-antigens. The paramount concern is to dampen this response so that tissue damage ceases. Immunosuppressive therapy is thus a critical element in a therapeutic regimen. Each disease discussion in this article has referred to immunosuppressive therapy. Some of the common immunosuppressive medications are listed in **Box 1**. Often a combination of these medications is used for optimum effect (eg, prednisone

---

Box 1
List of commonly used immunosuppressive drugs[a]

Azathioprine (Imuran)

Corticosteroids[b] (dexamethasone, prednisone, methylprednisolone)

Chlorambucil (Leukeran)

Cyclophosphamide (Cytoxan)

Cyclosporine (Sandimmune, Neoral)

Gold salts

Human intravenous immunoglobulin

[a] For specific use and dosage, see Nelson.[70]
[b] Immunosuppressive doses.

---

and azathioprine). The total therapy for each disease, however, is determined by the nature of the disease and the organ systems affected. For example, patients with IMHA in hemolytic crisis must be managed to control the anemia and stabilize the condition in conjunction with institution of the immunosuppressive therapy. Choice of drug and dosage is dependent on whether or not the object is to initiate remission, maintain remission, or rescue form acute crisis. The criteria and appropriate dosing information are presented in the textbook on internal medicine edited by Nelson and Couto.[11] Management of autoimmune skin diseases includes not only systemic immunosuppressive therapy but also topical and often systemic antimicrobial therapy that may be required.[32–35]

Some autoimmune diseases can be traced to the use of particular medications (such as a sufonamides and propylthiouracil).[68,69] In such cases, immunosuppressive therapy is coupled with discontinuation of the causative medication. The prognosis for clinical improvement and eventual discontinuation of the immunosuppressive therapy is good in these cases. Treatment of hyperthyroid cats with propylthiouracil causes a Coombs-positive and ANA-positive syndrome in some cats.[69] This lupus-like syndrome is characterized by lethargy, weight loss, lymphadenopathy, and anemia. In 1 study, more than half of a group of normal healthy cats treated with 6-propylthiouracil (150 mg daily) developed the syndrome. In the majority of the cats, the clinical and serologic signs resolved within 4 weeks of discontinuation of the medication.[68] Those cases for which there is no instigating cause (unfortunately, the majority of cases) are often held in remission by chronic low dose use of an immunosuppressive drug, such as prednisone.

SUMMARY

There are many autoimmune diseases recognized in humans; many of these have counterparts described in companion animals. The diseases discussed in this article do not constitute the entire spectrum of autoimmune disease in these species. They are the common and better-described diseases of dogs and cats that have a well-documented autoimmune etiology.

There are myriad autoimmune diseases that affect humans; it is likely that similar diseases yet unrecognized in companion animals will be characterized by astute clinicians in the future. The role of genetics in predisposition to autoimmunity is a common characteristic of these diseases in humans and animals. Likewise, the suggested role of environmental or infectious agents as instigators is another commonality between humans and the pets that share their environment.

REFERENCES

1. Figueroa-Vega N, Alfonso-Pérez M, Benedicto I, et al. Increased circulating pro-inflammatory cytokines and Th17 lymphocytes in Hashimoto's thyroiditis. J Clin Endocrinol Metab 2010;95(2):953–62.
2. Afzali B, Lombardi G, Lechler RI, et al. The role of T helper 17 (Th17) and regulatory T cells (Treg) in human organ transplantation and autoimmune disease. Clin Exp Immunol 2007;148(1):32–46.
3. Gaffen SL. The role of interleukin-17 in the pathogenesis of rheumatoid arthritis. Curr Rheumatol Rep 2009;11(5):365–70.
4. Bertolaccini ML, Hughes GRV, Khamashta MA. Systemic lupus erythematosus. In: Shoenfeld Y, Cervera R, Gershwin ME, editors. Diagnostic criteria in autoimmune diseases. New Jersey: Humana Press; 2008. p. 3–8.
5. Techner M, Krumbacher K, Doxiadis I, et al. Systemic lupus erythematosus in dogs: association to the major histocompatibility complex class I antigen DLA-A7. Clin Immunol Immunopathol 1990;55:255–62.
6. Fournel C, Chabanne L, Caux C, et al. Canine systemic lupus erythematosus. I: a study of 75 cases. Lupus 1992;1(3):133–9.
7. Monestier M, Novick KE, Karam ET, et al. Autoantibodies to histone, DNA, and nucleosome antigens in canine systemic lupus erythematousus. Clin Exp Immunol 1995;99:37–41.
8. Smee NM, Harkin KR, Wilkerson MJ. Measurement of serum antinuclear antibody titer in dogs with and without systemic lupus erythematosus: 120 cases (1997–2005). J Am Vet Med Assoc 2007;230(8):1180–3.
9. Aucoin DP, Rubin RL, Peterson ME, et al. Dose-dependent induction of anti-native DNA antibodies in cats by propylthiouracil. Arthritis Rheum. 1988;31(5):688–92.
10. Balch A, Mackin A. Canine immune-mediated hemolytic anemia: pathophysiology, clinical signs, and diagnosis [review]. Compend Contin Educ Vet 2007; 29(4):217–25.
11. Nelson RW. Anemia. In: Nelson RW, Couto CG, editors. Small animal internal medicine. 3rd edition. St Louis (MO): Mosby; 2003. p. 1162–4.
12. Kohn B, Weingart C, Eckmann V, et al. Primary immune-mediated hemolytic anemia in 19 cats: diagnosis, therapy, and outcome (1998–2004). J Vet Intern Med 2006;20(1):159–66.
13. Warman SM, Murray JK, Ridyard A, et al. Pattern of Coombs' test reactivity has diagnostic significance in dogs with immune-mediated haemolytic anaemia. J Small Anim Pract 2008;49(10):525–30.
14. Kennedy LJ, Barnes A, Ollier WE, et al. Association of a common dog leucocyte antigen class II haplotype with canine primary immune-mediated haemolytic anemia. Tissue Antigens 2006;68(6):502–8.
15. Whelan MF, O'Toole TE, Chan DL, et al. Use of human immunoglobulin in addition to glucocorticoids for the initial treatment of dogs with immune-mediated hemolytic anemia. J Vet Emerg CritCare (San Antonio) 2009;19(2):158–64.
16. Goggs R, Boag AK, Chan DL. Concurrent immune-mediated haemolytic anaemia and severe thrombocytopenia in 21 dogs. Vet Rec 2008;163(11): 323–7.
17. Dircks BH, Schuberth HJ, Mischke R. Underlying diseases and clinicopathologic variables of thrombocytopenic dogs with and without platelet-bound antibodies

detected by use of a flow cytometric assay: 83 cases (2004–2006). J Am Vet Med Assoc 2009;235(8):960–6.

18. Horgan JE, Roberts BK, Schermerhorn T. Splenectomy as an adjunctive treatment for dogs with immune-mediated hemolytic anemia: ten cases (2003–2006). J Vet Emerg Crit Care (San Antonio) 2009;19(3):254–61.

19. Bianco D, Armstrong PJ, Washabau RJ. Treatment of severe immune-mediated thrombocytopenia with human IV immunoglobulin in 5 dogs. J Vet Intern Med 2007;21(4):694–9.

20. Cortese L, Sica M, Piantedosi D, et al. Secondary immune-mediated thrombocytopenia in dogs naturally infected by *Leishmania infantum*. Vet Rec 2009;164(25): 778–82.

21. Vargo CL, Taylor SM, Haines DM. Immune mediated neutropenia and thrombocytopenia in 3 giant schnauzers. Can Vet J 2007;8(11):1159–63.

22. Rocchi R, Rose NR. Hashimoto thyroiditis. In: Shoenfeld Y, Cervera R, Gershwin ME, editors. Diagnostic criteria in autoimmune diseases. New Jersey: Humana Press; 2008. p. 217–20.

23. Nelson RW. Disorders of the thyroid gland. In: Nelson RW, Couto CG, editors. Small animal internal medicine. 3rd edition. St Louis (MO): Mosby; 2003. p. 691–4.

24. Kennedy LJ, Quarmby S, Happ GM, et al. Association of canine hypothyroidism with a common major histocompatibility complex DLA class II allele. Tissue Antigens 2006;68(1):82–6.

25. Catchpole B, Kennedy LJ, Davison LJ, et al. Canine diabetes mellitus: from phenotype to genotype. J Small Anim Pract 2008;49(1):4–10.

26. Ferm K, Björnerfeldt S, Karlsson A, et al. Prevalence of diagnostic characteristics indicating canine autoimmune lymphocytic thyroiditis in giant schnauzer and hovawart dogs. J Small Anim Pract 2009;50(4):176–9.

27. Choi EW, Shin IS, Bhang DH, et al. Hormonal change and cytokine mRNA expression in peripheral blood mononuclear cells during the development of canine autoimmune thyroiditis. Clin Exp Immunol 2006;146(1):101–8.

28. Nelson RW. Disorders of the endocrine pancreas. In: Nelson RW, Couto CG, editors. Small animal internal medicine. 3rd edition. St Louis (MO): Mosby; 2003. p. 729–33, 749–52.

29. Hoenig M, Reusch C, Peterson ME. Beta cell and insulin antibodies in treated and untreated diabetic cats. Vet Immunol Immunopathol 2000;77(1–2): 93–102.

30. Petersen JS, Hejnaes KR, Moody A, et al. Detection of GAD65 antibodies in diabetes and other autoimmune diseases using a simple radioligand assay. Diabetes 1994;43(3):459–67.

31. Davison LJ, Weenink SM, Christie MR, et al. Autoantibodies to GAD65 and IA-2 in canine diabetes mellitus. Vet Immunol Immunopathol 2008;126(1–2):83–90.

32. Medleau L, Hnilica KA. Discoid lupus. In: Small animal dermatology. 2nd edition. St. Louis (MO): Saunders-Elsevier; 2006. p. 204.

33. Medleau L, Hnilica KA. Pemphigus foliaceous. In: Small animal dermatology. 2nd edition. St. Louis (MO): Saunders-Elsevier; 2006. p. 190.

34. Medleau L, Hnilica KA. Pemphigus vulgaris. In: Small animal dermatology. 2nd edition. St. Louis (MO): Saunders-Elsevier; 2006. p. 199.

35. Medleau L, Hnilica KA. Bullous pemphigoid. In: Small animal dermatology. 2nd edition. St. Louis (MO): Saunders-Elsevier; 2006. p. 202.

36. Olivry T, Dunston SM, Walker RH, et al. Investigations on the nature and pathogenicity of circulating antikeratinocyte antibodies in dogs with pemphigus foliaceus. Vet Dermatol 2009;20(1):42–50.

37. Nishifuji K, Olivry T, Ishii K, et al. IgG autoantibodies directed against desmoglein 3 cause dissociation of keratinocytes in canine pemphigus vulgaris and paraneoplastic pemphigus. Vet Immunol Immunopathol 2007;117(3–4):209–21.

38. Nishifuji K, Yoshida-Yamakita K, Iwasaki T. A canine pemphigus foliaceus case showing parallel relationship of disease activity and titer of serum anti-keratinocyte cell surface antibodies. J Vet Med Sci 2005;67(9):943–5.

39. Shelton GD. Myasthenia gravis and disorders of neuromuscular transmission [review]. Vet Clin North Am Small Anim Pract 2002;32(1):189–206, vii.

40. Couturier J, Huynh M, Boussarie D, et al. Autoimmune myasthenia gravis in a ferret. J Am Vet Med Assoc 2009;235(12):1462–6.

41. Shelton GD, Schule A, Kass PH. Risk factors for acquired myasthenia gravis in dogs: 1,154 cases (1991–1995). J Am Vet Med Assoc 1997;211(11):1428–31.

42. Uchida K, Awamura Y, Nakamura T, et al. Thymoma and multiple thymic cysts in a dog with acquired myasthenia gravis. J Vet Med Sci 2002;64(7):637–40.

43. Wood SL, Rosenstein DS, Bebchuk T. Myasthenia gravis and thymoma in a dog. Vet Rec 2001;148(18):573–4.

44. Day MJ. Review of thymic pathology in 30 cats and 36 dogs [review]. J Small Anim Pract 1997;38(9):393–403.

45. Shelton GD, Ho M, Kass PH. Risk factors for acquired myasthenia gravis in cats: 105 cases (1986–1998). J Am Vet Med Assoc 2000;216(1):55–7.

46. Nelson RW. Disorders of peripheral nerves and the neuromuscular junction. In: Nelson RW, Couto CG, editors. Small Animal internal medicine. 3rd edition. Mosby; 2003. p. 1059–61.

47. Luo J, Lindstrom J. Antigenic structure of the human muscle nicotinic acetylcholine receptor main immunogenic region. J Mol Neurosci 2010;40(1–2):217–20.

48. Heuser W. Canine rheumatoid arthritis. Can Vet J 1980;21(11):314–6.

49. Lubberts E, van den Berg WB. Potential of modulatory cytokines in the rheumatoid arthritis process. Drug News Perspect 2001;14(9):517–22.

50. Moreland LW. The role of cytokines in rheumatoid arthritis: inhibition of cytokines in therapeutic trials. Drugs Today (Barc) 1999;35(4–5):309–19.

51. Jazayeri JA, Carroll GJ, Vernallis AB. Interleukin-6 subfamily cytokines and rheumatoid arthritis: role of antagonists. Int Immunopharmacol 2010;10(1):1–8.

52. Hegemann N, Wondimu A, Ullrich K, et al. Synovial MMP-3 and TIMP-1 levels and their correlation with cytokine expression in canine rheumatoid arthritis. Vet Immunol Immunopathol 2003;91(3–4):199–204.

53. Ollier WE, Kennedy LJ, Thomson W, et al. Dog MHC alleles containing the human RA shared epitope confer susceptibility to canine rheumatoid arthritis. Immunogenetics 2001;53(8):669–73.

54. May C, Carter SD, Bell SC, et al. Immune responses to canine distemper virus in joint diseases of dogs. Br J Rheumatol 1994;33(1):27–31.

55. Bell SC, Carter SD, Bennett D. Canine distemper viral antigens and antibodies in dogs with rheumatoid arthritis. Res Vet Sci 1991;50(1):64–8.

56. Roush JK, Manley PA, Dueland RT. Rheumatoid arthritis subsequent to Borrelia burgdorferi infection in two dogs. J Am Vet Med Assoc 1989;195(7):951–3.

57. Angles JM, Famula TR, Pedersen NC. Uveodermatologic (VKH-like) syndrome in American Akita dogs is associated with an increased frequency of DQA1*00201. Tissue Antigens 2005;66(6):656–65.

58. Medleau L, Hnilica KA. Canine uveodermatologic syndrome (Vogt-Koyangi-Harada-like syndrome, VKH). In: Small animal dermatology. 2nd edition. St. Louis (MO): Saunders-Elsevier; 2006. p. 292.

59. Yamaki K, Ohono S. Animal models of Vogt-Koyanagi-Harada disease (sympathetic ophthalmia). Ophthalmic Res 2008;40(3–4):129–35.
60. Hansson-Hamlin H, Lilliehöök I, Trowald-Wigh G. Subgroups of canine antinuclear antibodies in relation to laboratory and clinical findings in immune-mediated disease. Vet Clin Pathol 2006;35(4):397–404.
61. Ginel PJ, Camacho S, Lucena R. Anti-histone antibodies in dogs with leishmaniasis and glomerulonephritis. Res Vet Sci 2008;85(3):510–4.
62. Smith BE, Tompkins MB, Breitschwerdt EB. Antinuclear antibodies can be detected in dog sera reactive to *Bartonella vinsonii* subsp. berkhoffii, *Ehrlichia canis*, or *Leishmania infantum* antigens. J Vet Intern Med 2004;18(1): 47–51.
63. Conrad K, Ittenson A, Reinhold D, et al. High sensitive detection of double-stranded DNA autoantibodies by a modified Crithidia luciliae immunofluorescence test. Ann N Y Acad Sci 2009;1173:180–5.
64. Welin Henriksson E, Hansson H, Karlsson-Parra A, et al. Autoantibody profiles in canine ANA-positive sera investigated by immunoblot and ELISA [review]. Vet Immunol Immunopathol 1998;61(2–4):157–70.
65. Hansson H, Karlsson-Parra A. Canine antinuclear antibodies: comparison of immunofluorescence staining patterns and precipitin reactivity. Acta Vet Scand 1999;40(3):205–12.
66. Hansson-Hamlin H, Rönnelid J. Detection of antinuclear antibodies by the Inno-Lia ANA update test in canine systemic rheumatic disease. Vet Clin Pathol 2009. [Epub ahead of print].
67. Warman SM, Murray JK, Ridyard A, et al. Pattern of Coombs' test reactivity has diagnostic significance in dogs with immune-mediated haemolytic anaemia. J Small Anim Pract 2008;49(10):525–30.
68. Aucoin DP, Peterson ME, Hurvitz AI, et al. Propylthiouracil-induced immune-mediated disease in the cat. J Pharmacol Exp Ther 1985;234(1):13–8.
69. Aucoin DP, Rubin RL, Peterson ME, et al. Dose-dependent induction of anti-native DNA antibodies in cats by propylthiouracil. Arthritis Rheum 1988;31(5):688–92.
70. Nelson RW. Immunosuppressive drugs. In: Nelson RW, Couto CG, editors. Small animal internal medicine. 3rd edition. St Louis (MO): Mosby; 2003. p. 1216–9.

Noninfectious Causes of Immunosuppression in Dogs and Cats

Craig A. Datz, DVM, MS

KEYWORDS

- Immunosuppression • Malnutrition • Vaccination
- Stress • Anesthesia • Aging

Diseases associated with immunosuppression or immune system deficiency are not common but when present can lead to decreased resistance to infection, debilitation, and other complications of illness. Components of the immune system may be functionally divided into humoral and cellular immunity, with some degree of overlap. Diagnostic evaluation of these immunologic functions is available in specialized research laboratories but not widely available to practitioners.[1] The basic approach to a patient suspected as having immunodeficiency starts with routine laboratory work, including a complete blood count and chemistry profile. More specific testing may involve measurements of antibody concentrations, lymphocyte phenotyping, and lymphocyte function testing.[1]

A variety of drugs, toxins, diseases, and procedures such as vaccination and anesthesia have been associated with immunosuppression in dogs and cats. The following information is taken from published scientific literature, with an emphasis on animal studies where available. As the review is not comprehensive, interested readers are encouraged to consult the references and current immunology resources to gain a greater understanding of the effects of these agents on the immune system.

NUTRITION

The effects of nutrition on the immune system continue to be investigated in human and veterinary medicine. Immune-enhancing, immunomodulating, and immunosuppressive diets, foods, supplements, and nutrients have been suggested, often with little or no clinical evidence.[2]

In a study of young beagle dogs, short-term dietary restriction led to decreases in levels of IgG and C3, antibody titers, lymphocyte counts, lymphocyte response to mitogens, neutrophil counts, and neutrophil chemotaxis.[3] Most of these immune markers improved after refeeding. In cats, short-term food deprivation caused

Department of Veterinary Medicine and Surgery, College of Veterinary Medicine, University of Missouri, 900 East Campus Drive, Columbia, MO 65211, USA
E-mail address: datzc@missouri.edu

Vet Clin Small Anim 40 (2010) 459–467
doi:10.1016/j.cvsm.2010.02.004   **vetsmall.theclinics.com**

decreased total leukocyte and lymphocyte counts, a change in the proportion of T cells (decreased CD4 to CD8 ratio), and decreased lymphocyte proliferation.[4] As in the canine study, most of these outcomes improved with refeeding. The concept is that dietary deficiency (decreased intake) of protein can cause immunosuppression but it is difficult to know for sure as the studies do not account for deficiency of vitamins and minerals as well.

Most of the knowledge pertaining to nutrition and immunity is derived from human and laboratory animal studies. Direct extrapolation to companion animals should not be assumed. The following are examples of nutrients that have been shown to be involved in immunodeficiency.

Protein and Amino Acid Balance

A deficiency of dietary protein intake leads to low concentrations of amino acids, which can result in immunosuppression and decreased resistance to infectious disease. Amino acids are involved in the activation of T and B cells, natural killer (NK) cells, and macrophages. They are also necessary for gene expression, lymphocyte proliferation, and the production of antibodies, cytokines, and other cytotoxic substances.[5] Arginine is necessary for lymphocyte development, and a deficiency leads to decreased number of B cells in secondary lymphoid organs. Aspartate and glutamate are involved in the metabolism and function of leukocytes as well as the proliferation of lymphocytes. Glutamate is a substrate for the synthesis of γ-aminobutyrate (GABA), which is present in macrophages and lymphocytes, and T cells express GABA receptors. A dietary deficiency of branched-chain amino acids decreases tumor cell lysis and increases susceptibility to infection. Glutamine supplementation enhances immunity in humans and animals, suggesting that a deficiency may lead to immunosuppression. Animal studies have shown that lysine deficiency decreases immunity. The sulfur-containing amino acids (methionine and cysteine) are necessary for T- and B-cell proliferation and function, and supplementation increases disease resistance in animals.[5] Taurine-deficient diets in cats lead to several adverse consequences, including atrophy of the spleen and lymph nodes, lymphopenia, and impaired oxidative burst by phagocytes.[2]

Lipids

Dietary fats and oils can influence immunity in a variety of ways.[2] Both the content and composition of fatty acids in the diet have been shown to be immunomodulating. When studied in vitro, polyunsaturated fatty acids (PUFAs) inhibit lymphocyte proliferation and NK cell activity, decrease secretion of cytokines, and lead to a shift away from a helper 1 T cell response.[6] Human and animal studies have demonstrated immunosuppressive effects of long-chain PUFAs at high doses and have been used to treat immune-mediated conditions such as rheumatoid arthritis. However, evidence is equivocal and sometimes contradictory, depending on subjects, experimental conditions, and measured outcomes.[7]

Minerals

Adequate dietary copper intake is important for maintaining immune responses. Deficiencies can lead to decreased antibody production and cell-mediated immunity, with an increased susceptibility to infection.[2] Zinc deficiency is associated with lymphopenia, thymic atrophy, reductions in lymphocyte proliferation, NK and CD4 cell activity, and decreased chemotaxis of neutrophils. Dietary iron deficiency or increased iron loss can lead to a decrease in T cell responses, cytokine and antibody production, and phagocytic activity.[2] Selenium deficiency impairs lymphocyte proliferation, antibody production, and neutrophil chemotaxis.[8]

Vitamins

Several dietary vitamin deficiencies can lead to immunosuppression. Vitamin A has been widely studied in humans and animals, and dietary deficiency causes abnormalities in epithelial and mucosal surfaces (innate immunity), impaired neutrophil and NK cell function, decreases in number and function of B cells, and increased risk of infection.[2,9] Vitamin E at low dietary levels in dogs caused a decrease in lymphocyte proliferation.[10] B complex vitamins, especially pyridoxine, may impair both humoral and cell-mediated immunity if deficient.[2]

VACCINATION

Dogs and cats have long been suspected to experience transient immunosuppression after the administration of vaccines, especially modified live products. Clinical observations of infectious disease occurring within days of vaccination led to the hypothesis of vaccine-induced immunosuppression.[11,12] A limited number of studies, with varying methodology and outcomes, have been reported in dogs.

Eight adult dogs were vaccinated with modified live virus (MLV) canine parvovirus vaccine, and lymphocyte blastogenesis response was measured at 6 time points up to a month later.[13] The response to concanavalin A (ConA) was suppressed in 3 of 8 dogs. In a larger study involving 92 puppies (3–11 months of age), both monovalent and polyvalent vaccines were studied. Measurements of leukocyte counts, chemiluminescence, and lymphocyte blastogenesis were performed up to 2 weeks later.[14] There were no effects on leukocytes except decreases in lymphocyte counts on days 5 and 7 with several of the polyvalent vaccines. The lymphocyte response to phytohemagglutinin (PHA) was transiently suppressed with 2 of the polyvalent vaccines.

In contrast to these studies, a report of puppies and adult dogs showed an increase in lymphocyte blastogenesis response to PHA.[15] Total leukocyte and lymphocyte counts were reduced at day 7. Another study of the effect of vaccination on lymphocyte response to ConA in association with surgery showed a nonsignificant slight decrease.[16]

Despite the apparent reduction in immunity after MLV vaccination as determined by lymphocyte stimulation studies, animals typically respond with increases in antibody titers. Acute onset of infectious disease is rare in recently vaccinated dogs and cats, which suggests that any immunosuppression is transient and clinically insignificant. One explanation is that the balance between cell-mediated and humoral (antibody-mediated) immunity transiently shifts after vaccination. This was demonstrated in a study of 33 adult dogs (age, 2–13.5 years) receiving routine annual polyvalent vaccines.[17] Outcomes measured before and 2 weeks after vaccination included white cell counts and differentials, levels of cytokines (interleukin-1 [IL-1], IL-2, interferon-γ [IFN-γ], tumor necrosis factor α), and markers of humoral response (IgG, complement system activity) and cell-mediated response (lymphocyte proliferation to PHA, NK cell activity, bactericidal activity, neopterin concentration). The results indicated increases in levels of cytokines, IgG, and complement activity and decreases in lymphocyte response and levels of neopterin. Therefore, a transient shift in the immune response from cell-mediated to humoral seems to be more likely than a reduction in immune system function. When vaccination is performed in healthy animals, concerns about immunosuppression seem unfounded.

ANESTHESIA

Immunosuppression resulting from anesthesia has been reported, but research is complicated by confounding factors such as stress from surgical trauma, pain, hypothermia, hypotension, and direct effects of anesthetic drugs.[18] Any immunomo-dulating effects of anesthesia are likely to be overwhelmed by the neuroendocrine stress response.[19]

Several studies concerning potential immunosuppression associated with anes-thesia have been performed in dogs and cats. Adult female dogs undergoing ovario-hysterectomy were anesthetized with xylazine and ketamine alone or followed by halothane and nitrous oxide.[20] A transient depression in phagocytosis compared with controls was noted up to 4 hours postsurgery but resolved by 24 hours. Lympho-cyte stimulation in response to mitogens was reduced immediately after surgery and persisted throughout the observation period of 7 days. In another study, young and older adult dogs were vaccinated from 10 days prior up to 3 days after various surgical procedures.[16] No significant differences in antibody titers or lymphocyte blastogene-sis were observed compared with control dogs (no anesthesia or surgery performed). In feral cats 4 months of age or older, vaccination at the time of anesthesia and spay/neuter surgery did not reduce antibody responses.[21] The drugs used in that study included tiletamine, zolazepam, ketamine, xylazine, and isoflurane, and yohimbine was used as a partial reversal agent. Another study in specific-pathogen-free kittens showed no difference in antibody response to vaccines given at or within 1 week of the time of neutering with the use of butorphanol and isoflurane.[22] Immunity, as measured by antibody titers after vaccination, was not affected by general anesthesia or surgical stress in these studies.

DRUGS

Several medications are used in human and veterinary medicine to suppress or modu-late the immune system. These agents are specifically used to treat inflammatory, immune-mediated, and neoplastic diseases in dogs and cats, and side effects result-ing from immunosuppression should be monitored during and after therapy. The following is a brief review of some of the drug properties, mechanisms, and effects.

Glucocorticoids

These agents are often a first-line treatment for immune-mediated diseases. A wide range of immune cells is affected, but the current understanding of pharmacokinetic and immunologic effects is limited. Most of the evidence is anecdotal, empiric, based on in vitro studies, or extrapolated from other species.[23] In dogs, glucocorticoids reduced the proportion of certain phenotypic markers on lymphocytes and induced apoptosis in vitro.[24] The effects observed with neutrophils include decreased chemo-taxis and phagocytosis, suppression of antibody-dependent cellular cytotoxicity, and depressed bactericidal activity. Likewise, macrophages have decreased chemotaxis and phagocytosis as well as reductions in antigen processing and IL-1 production. Lymphocytes show reductions in proliferation and lymphokine production, decreased T-cell responses, impaired T cell–mediated cytotoxicity, and reduced IL-2 production.[25]

Azathioprine

This drug suppresses activated lymphocytes and inhibits proliferation of macro-phages.[25] Cell-mediated and humoral immunity are affected.[26]

Cyclosporine

This calcineurin inhibitor acts on T cells to block production of IL-2 and IFN-γ, which suppresses T_H1 response.[25]

Cyclophosphamide and Chlorambucil

The drugs cyclophosphamide and chlorambucil are nitrogen mustard chemotherapeutic agents that impair B and T cell responses by blocking cell division and cytokine production, such as IFN γ. Macrophage function is suppressed, B cells are destroyed, and antibody production is decreased.[25,27]

Methotrexate

Methotrexate is a folic acid analogue that inhibits purine and thymidylate synthesis, which leads to decreased antibody production.[28]

Mycophenolate

This drug also inhibits purine synthesis, suppressing lymphocyte proliferation and antibody production by B cells.[26,27]

Leflunomide

Leflunomide is an immunosuppressant that was originally used to prevent tissue rejection in renal transplants.[29] Pyrimidine synthesis and tyrosine kinases are inhibited, leading to decreased T- and B-cell responsiveness.[26]

STRESS AND EXERCISE

Physiologic stress may contribute to immunosuppression, although research is limited in small animals. Examples in large animals include shipping fever in cattle and early weaning in piglets, where disease resistance is apparently decreased by stress.[30] Among the proposed mechanisms are decreases in T-cell responses, NK cell activity, and production of IL-2. One report of African wild dogs attributed loss of the population studied to the stress of handling, including capture, immobilization, vaccination, blood sampling, and applying radiotelemetry collars.[31] Immunosuppression leading to viral infection was hypothesized to contribute to the extinction of this group.

Exercise may lead to decreased immunity. Conditioned Alaskan sled dogs were exercised for 5 consecutive days, and blood was collected for routine work and analyzed before the study and during each day of the study.[32] Mean serum globulin concentrations were low at rest and progressively decreased throughout the exercise period. One explanation was a possible immunosuppressive effect of the exercise, but increased catabolism may have played a role. A study in purpose-bred laboratory beagles failed to show significant effects of mild exercise on measures of immune status.[33]

ENDOCRINOPATHIES

Some diseases of the endocrine system have deleterious effects on the immune system. For example, humans with diabetes mellitus (DM) have higher rates and severity of infections, which are correlated with abnormalities in cell-mediated immunity and phagocytic function.[34] Less is known about immunosuppression in small animals, but disorders of the thymus and the thyroid along with diabetes and cortisol excess have been proposed as causes of immunodeficiency.[35]

A group of inbred Weimaraner puppies were found to have a wasting disease characterized by unthriftiness, emaciation, and persistent infections.[36] Several puppies were found to have atrophic or hypoplastic thymus glands, depressed lymphocyte blastogenic response, growth hormone (GH) deficiency, and a positive response to injection of thymosin (a thymic hormone involved in T-lymphocyte maturation). A later study demonstrated a clinical response to either thymosin or GH therapy, but lymphocyte blastogenesis was not improved.[37]

Dogs with DM may be predisposed to infections. In one retrospective study, 21% of dogs with DM were diagnosed with urinary tract infection through aerobic bacterial culture.[38] Another retrospective study found that dogs with DM and skin disease had a high prevalence of bacterial skin infection (84%) and yeast dermatitis (42%).[39] However, because of concurrent diseases such as allergy and use of corticosteroid medication in some dogs, a direct correlation between infection and DM could not be made. One proposed mechanism for increased infections is decreased neutrophil adherence, which was demonstrated in poorly controlled diabetic dogs.[40] However, the clinical significance is unknown.

An excess of circulating cortisol, either exogenous through medications or endogenous as seen in hyperadrenocorticism, may be immunosuppressive (see Drugs section).

RADIATION

Ultraviolet radiation from excessive exposure to the sun may be immunosuppressive in humans.[41] Animals are typically more resistant to solar damage because of hair coat, pigmentation, and other protective factors.[42] Photoimmunologic suppression induced by UV radiation includes changes in antigen-presenting cells in the skin and activation of regulatory T cells.[43]

Radiation exposure from imaging studies or radiation therapy can lead to a reduction in lymphocytes and adverse effects on lymphoid tissue.[44] Total-body irradiation inhibits the immune response to new antigens, whereas partial-body therapy has only a limited effect.

TRAUMA

Animals that are injured or critically ill may experience immunosuppression caused by tissue damage. Evidence in laboratory animals suggests that antigen-presenting cell and T-cell dysfunction along with endogenous "danger signals" released after trauma lead to increased risk of infection and other complications.[45] Cytokines produced by macrophages and damaged tissues can affect the immune system. The functions of macrophages, neutrophils, and T cells are impaired, but B cells and antibody responses may be normal.[30]

TOXINS

Chemical and environmental toxins have been linked with immunosuppression in human and animal studies. Little is known about the effects of toxins on the immune system of dogs and cats, but monitoring may be indicated in cases of exposure. Suspected immunosuppressive toxins include insecticides, herbicides, fungicides, halogenated cyclic hydrocarbons, heavy metals, and mycotoxins.[46] Detrimental effects on both cell-mediated and humoral immune responses have been reported in various animal species. Mycotoxins in particular may contaminate commercial pet food, leading to acute and chronic toxicity, including immunosuppression.[47,48]

AGE

Age-related alterations in immune function, or immunosenescence, have been documented in humans and rodents. The incidence and severity of infections, autoimmune diseases, and neoplasia seen in older humans may have a basis in immunosuppression, although physiologic effects of aging and genetics play major roles.[49]

In dogs, a life span study of Labrador retrievers has yielded valuable information on changes in immune system markers over time.[50] In a group of 23 dogs studied from age 4 to 11.5 years, some markers of immune response decreased over time. Mitogen-stimulated lymphocyte proliferation measured semiannually significantly declined, and the percentage of B lymphocytes were lower as dogs aged. No changes in NK cell activity or phagocytic activity of polymorphonuclear leukocytes were observed. An earlier cross-sectional study in the same population of dogs showed similar results.[51] In another cross-sectional study of client-owned young and old dogs, lymphocyte proliferation in response to mitogens was decreased in the older group.[52] The implication is that immunosenescence can be measured and may be predictive of survival. Using Cox proportional hazards modeling, earlier death in the Labrador population was associated with lower lymphoproliferative responses; fewer total lymphocytes, T cells, CD4 cells, and CD8 cells; and lower CD8 cell and higher B-cell percentages.[53] In the future, the ability to identify trends toward decreased immunity and possible treatment may lead to longer, healthier life spans.

SUMMARY

Immunosuppression has been identified in human and animal studies to be a result of trauma and disease, therapeutic drugs, toxins, stress, and medical procedures such as anesthesia. Lifelong issues such as nutrition, stress, and exercise also have effects on the immune system. Veterinarians should be aware of the potential for immunodeficiency when dealing with both healthy and diseased patients. As the recognition and treatment of immunosuppression can be difficult, exposure to these noninfectious causes should be minimized or avoided if possible.

REFERENCES

1. Day MJ. Immunodiagnostic tests of immune function. Clinical immunology. Sydney (Australia): University of Sydney, Centre for Veterinary Education; 2008. p. 207–13.
2. Saker KE. Nutrition and immune function. Vet Clin North Am Small Anim Pract 2006;36:1199–224.
3. Dionigi R, Zonta A, Dominioni L, et al. The effects of total parenteral nutrition on immunodepression due to malnutrition. Ann Surg 1977;185:467–74.
4. Frietag KA, Saker KE, Thomas E, et al. Acute starvation and subsequent refeeding affect lymphocyte subsets and proliferation in cats. J Nutr 2000;130:2444–9.
5. Li P, Yin L, Li D, et al. Amino acids and immune function. Br J Nutr 2007;98: 237–52.
6. Stulnig TM. Immunomodulation by polyunsaturated fatty acids; mechanisms and effects. Int Arch Allergy Immunol 2003;132:310–21.
7. Fritsche K. Fatty acids as modulators of the immune response. Annu Rev Nutr 2006;26:45–73.
8. Beckett GJ, Arthur JR, Miller SM, et al. Selenium. In: Hughes DA, Darlington LG, Bendich A, editors. Diet and human immune function. Totowa (NJ): Humana Press; 2004. p. 217–40.
9. Semba RD. Vitamin A. In: Hughes DA, Darlington LG, Bendich A, editors. Diet and human immune function. Totowa (NJ): Humana Press; 2004. p. 105–31.
10. Meydani SN, Hayek MG, Wu D, et al. Vitamin E and immune reponse in aged dogs. In: Reinhart GA, Carey DP, editors. Recent advances in canine and feline

nutrition. Proceedings of the Iams 1998 Nutrition Symposium. Wilmington (OH): Orange Frazer Press; 1998. p. 295–303.

11. Bestetti G, Fatzer R, Fankhauser R. Encephalitis following vaccination against distemper and infectious hepatitis in the dog. Acta Neuropathol 1978;43:69–75.

12. Kesel LM, Neil DH. Combined MLV canine parvovirus vaccine: immunosuppression with infective shedding. Vet Med Small Anim Clin 1983;5:687–91.

13. Mastro JM, Axthelm M, Mathes LE, et al. Repeated suppression of lymphocyte blastogenesis following vaccinations of CPV-immune dogs with modified-live CPV vaccines. Vet Microbiol 1986;12:201–11.

14. Phillips TR, Jensen JL, Rubino MJ, et al. Effects of vaccines on the canine immune system. Can J Vet Res 1989;53:154–60.

15. Miyamoto T, Taura Y, Une S, et al. Changes in blastogenic responses of lymphocytes and delayed type hypersensitivity responses after vaccination in dogs. J Vet Med Sci 1992;54:945–50.

16. Miyamoto T, Taura Y, Une S, et al. Immunological responses after vaccination pre- and post-surgery in dogs. J Vet Med Sci 1995;57:29–32.

17. Strasser A, May B, Teltscher A, et al. Immune modulation following immunization with polyvalent vaccines in dogs. Vet Immun Immunopathol 2003;94:113–21.

18. Kona-Boun JJ, Silim A, Troncy E. Immunologic aspects of veterinary anesthesia and analgesia. J Am Vet Med Assoc 2005;226:355–63.

19. Galley HF, DiMatteo MA, Webster NR. Immunomodulation by anaesthetic, sedative and analgesic agents: does it matter? Intensive Care Med 2001;26:267–74.

20. Mojzisova J, Hromada R, Valocky I, et al. Effect of ovariohysterectomy on canine postsurgical leukocyte function. Acta Vet Hung 2003;51:219–27.

21. Fischer SM, Quest CM, Dubovi EJ, et al. Response of feral cats to vaccination at the time of neutering. J Am Vet Med Assoc 2007;230:52–8.

22. Reese MJ, Patterson EV, Tucker SJ, et al. Effects of anesthesia and surgery on serologic responses to vaccination in kittens. J Am Vet Med Assoc 2008;233:116–21.

23. Day MJ. Immunotherapy I and II. Clinical immunology. Sydney (Australia): University of Sydney, Centre for Veterinary Education; 2008. p. 31–45.

24. Ammersbach MAG, Kruth SA, Sears W, et al. The effect of glucocorticoids on canine lymphocyte marker expression and apoptosis. J Vet Intern Med 2006; 20:1166–71.

25. Tizard IR. Veterinary immunology. St Louis (MO): Saunders Elsevier; 2009. p. 481–6.

26. Gregory CR. Immunosuppressive agents. In: Bonagura JD, editor. Kirk's current veterinary therapy XIV. St Louis (MO): Saunders Elsevier; 2009. p. 257–8.

27. Papich MG. Immunosuppressive drugs and cyclosporine. In: Riviere JE, Papich MG, editors. Veterinary pharmacology and therapeutics. 9th edition. Ames (IA): Wiley-Blackwell; 2009. p. 1233–46.

28. Coppoc GL. Chemotherapy of neoplastic diseases. In: Riviere JE, Papich MG, editors. Veterinary pharmacology and therapeutics. 9th edition. Ames (IA): Wiley-Blackwell; 2009. p. 1205–31.

29. McChesney LP, Xiao F, Sankary HN, et al. An evaluation of leflunomide in the canine renal transplantation model. Transplantation 1994;57:1717–22.

30. Tizard IR. Veterinary immunology. St Louis (MO): Saunders Elsevier; 2009. p. 473–9.

31. Burrows R, Hofer H, East ML. Population dynamics, intervention and survival in African wild dogs (Lycaon pictus). Proc Biol Sci 1995;262:235–45.

32. McKenzie EC, Jose-Cunilleras E, Hinchcliff KW, et al. Serum chemistry alterations in Alaskan sled dogs during five successive days of prolonged endurance exercise. J Am Vet Med Assoc 2007;230:1486–92.

33. Clark JD, Rager DR, Crowell-Davis S, et al. Housing and exercise of dogs: effects on behavior, immune function, and cortisol concentration. Lab Anim Sci 1997; 47(5):500–10.
34. Powers AC. Diabetes mellitus. In: Fauci AS, Braunwald E, Kasper DL, et al, editors. Harrison's principles of internal medicine. 17th edition. New York: McGraw Hill; 2008. p. 2292–3.
35. Greco DS, Harpold LM. Immunity and the endocrine system. Vet Clin North Am Small Anim Pract 1994;24:765–82.
36. Roth JA, Lomax LG, Altszuler N, et al. Thymic abnormalities and growth hormone deficiency in dogs. Am J Vet Res 1980;41:1256–62.
37. Roth JA, Kaeberle ML, Grier RK, et al. Improvement in clinical condition and thymus morphologic features associated with growth hormone treatment of immunodeficient dogs. Am J Vet Res 1984;45:1151–5.
38. Hess RS, Saunders HM, Van Winkle TJ, et al. Concurrent disorders in dogs with diabetes mellitus: 221 cases (1993–1998). J Am Vet Med Assoc 2000;217: 1166–73.
39. Peikes H, Morris DO, Hess RS. Dermatologic disorders in dogs with diabetes mellitus: 45 cases (1986–2000). J Am Vet Med Assoc 2001;219(2):203–8.
40. Latimer KS, Mahaffey EA. Neutrophil adherence and movement in poorly and well-controlled diabetic dogs. Am J Vet Res 1984;45:1498–500.
41. Norval M, McLoone P, Lesiak A, et al. The effect of chronic ultraviolet radiation on the human immune system. Photochem Photobiol 2008;84:19–28.
42. Scott DW, Miller WH, Griffin CE. Environmental skin diseases. In: Muller & Kirk's small animal dermatology. Philadelphia: WB Saunders; 2001. p. 1073–81.
43. Leitenberger J, Jacobe HT, Cruz PD. Photoimmunology—illuminating the immune system through photobiology. Semin Immunopathol 2007;29:65–70.
44. Hall EJ, Giaccia AJ. Clinical response of normal tissues. In: Radiobiology for the radiologist. Philadelphia: Lippincott Williams & Wilkins; 2006. p. 337.
45. Flohe SB, Flohe S, Schade FU. Deterioration of the immune system after trauma: signals and cellular mechanisms. Innate Immun 2008;14:333–44.
46. Cabassi E. The immune system and exposure to xenobiotics in animals. Vet Res Commun 2007;31(S1):115–20.
47. Oswald IP, Marin DE, Bouhet S, et al. Immunotoxicological risk of mycotoxins for domestic animals. Food Addit Contam 2005;22:354–60.
48. Boermans HJ, Leung MC. Mycotoxins and the pet food industry: toxicological evidence and risk assessment. Int J Food Microbiol 2007;119:95–102.
49. Fulop T, Hirokawa K, Mocchegiani E, et al. The immune system in the elderly. In: Karasek M, editor. Aging and age-related diseases: the basics. Hauppauge (NY): Nova Science Publishers; 2006. p. 173–96.
50. Greeley EH, Ballam JM, Harrison JM, et al. The influence of age and gender on the immune system: a longitudinal study in Labrador Retriever dogs. Vet Immunol Immunopathol 2001;82:57–71.
51. Greeley EH, Kealy RD, Ballam JM, et al. The influence of age on the canine immune system. Vet Immunol Immunopathol 1996;55:1–10.
52. HogenEsch H, Thompson S, Dunham A, et al. Effect of age on immune parameters and the immune response of dogs to vaccines: a cross-sectional study. Vet Immunol Immunopathol 2004;97:77–85.
53. Lawler DF, Larson BE, Ballam JM, et al. Diet restriction and ageing in the dog: major observations over two decades. Br J Nutr 2008;99:793–805.

Diagnostic Assays for Immunologic Diseases in Small Animals

Stephen A. Kania, PhD

KEYWORDS

• Immunologic diseases • Small animals • Diagnostic assays

Several tests are available for the diagnosis of immunologic disorders with varying availability. The tests are categorized into two groups, those that examine function and those that measure physical parameters such as cell numbers or immunoglobulin concentrations. Functional tests generally are less available because of issues of cell viability that affect storage and transportation.

LYMPHOCYTE PROLIFERATION/BLASTOGENESIS
Test of Lymphocyte Responsiveness

Lymphocytes are placed in short-term culture and stimulated with antigen or mitogen. Antigen will stimulate only a small proportion of lymphocytes, those with epitope-specific receptors. Mitogens, such as the plant lectins concanavalin A (ConA)[1] and phytohemagglutinin (PHA) bind to cell membrane glycoproteins including T-cell receptor complex and are broadly reactive with T-cells. Lipopolysaccharide targets B cells. Anti-CD3 targets T-cells by cross-linking T-cell receptors. Stimulated lympho-cytes respond with an increase in nucleic acid synthesis and cell proliferation. Response to mitogen is a measure of the capability of lymphocytes to become acti-vated and is associated with their ability to respond, in vivo, to antigenic stimulation. To measure this, lymphocytes are cultured for 48 hours with stimulant; tritiated thymi-dine then is added, and cells are harvested after a total of approximately 60 hours in culture. Incorporation of tritiated thymidine into the DNA of stimulated lymphocytes is measured using liquid scintillation counters. Tests using nonradioactive reagents are also available. Lipophilic fluorescent dyes include carboxyfluorescein diacetate succi-nimidyl ester (CFSE)[2] and 3-(4,5-dimethylthiazol-2-yl)-2,5-diphenyl tetrazolium bromide MTT.[3] CFSE labels lymphocyte membranes, and as the cells divide, each daughter cell contains half as much dye. Flow cytometry is used to enumerate the number of cells in each division class. Thus the number of cycles of cellular replication can be determined. The MTT assay is a colorimetric test based on the reduction of

Department of Comparative Medicine, College of Veterinary Medicine, University of Tennessee, 2407 River Drive, Knoxville, TN 37849, USA
E-mail address: skania@utk.edu

Vet Clin Small Anim 40 (2010) 469–472
doi:10.1016/j.cvsm.2010.03.001
0195-5616/10/$ – see front matter © 2010 Elsevier Inc. All rights reserved.

vetsmall.theclinics.com

yellow tetrazolium salt to insoluble purple crystals when it is metabolized. The crystals are solubilized with detergent, and the quantity of purple dye is measured with an enzyme-linked immunosorbent assay (ELISA) reader. There is a linear relationship between absorbance and the number of cells enabling a measurement of cell proliferation. Cytokines also are used to measure lymphocyte response to stimulation. This is accomplished with reverse transcription real-time polymerase chain reaction (PCR) for mRNA transcripts or ELISA to directly measure cytokines. For mRNA measurement, interferon (IFN)-gamma and interleukin (IL)-4 often are measured. IFN-gamma, IL-6, IL-10, and TNF-gamma quantitative ELISA kits are available for the dog from R&D Systems (Minneapolis, MN, USA). Real-time PCR primers and probes can be purchased from Applied Biosystems (Foster City, CA, USA), and primer assays for canine IFN-gamma, IL-4, IL-10, and transforming growth factor-beta are available from Qiagen (Valencia, CA, USA) and can be used with SYBR green.[4]

COMPLEMENT HEMOLYTIC ACTIVITY

Complement deposition is important for opsonization or direct destruction of microorganisms. Available tests for complement components are limited in companion animals. A test for total hemolytic activity can aid in the diagnosis of a functional complement deficiency. For this test, erythrocytes are coated with antibody, and complement-preserved patient serum is added in the presence of gelatin-veronal buffer. Complement-mediated lysis is determined by measuring the release of hemoglobin from the erythrocytes by spectrophotometry. This assay is used for research purposes for the cat[5] and dog[6] but is not readily available from commercial diagnostic laboratories. Use of the test is restricted because of the requirement to preserve complement activity, which includes shipment on dry ice and special storage.

ANTINUCLEAR ANTIBODY TEST

The antinuclear antibody test (ANA) detects antibodies reactive with nuclear components of cells. The ANA test is performed by incubating patient sera with a cell substrate, such as rat liver or mouse kidney cells. Fluorescein conjugated anti-IgG or anti-IgM detecting antibody, corresponding to the patient species, is added. Bound antibody is detected by the presence of fluorescence as observed with the use of a fluorescence microscope.

COOMBS TEST

The Coombs test is used to detect antibody and complement bound to the surface of erythrocytes. These antibodies may be directed against erythrocyte antigens or, in the case of secondary immune mediated hemolytic anemia (IMHA), against foreign antigen deposited on the surface of the cells as a result of infection or drug treatment. These components can mediate erythrocyte destruction and lead to IMHA. The test uses Coombs reagent consisting of host species-specific antibodies directed against IgG, IgM, and the third component of complement (C3). Washed erythrocytes are incubated with Coombs reagent at 37 C and 4 C and then checked for agglutination. The traditional test has been found to have a sensitivity of only about 60%.[7,8] Recently Warman and colleagues[7] demonstrated the advantage of using the individual components of Coombs reagent to achieve greater sensitivity. Alternative methods include enzyme-linked antiglobulin tests and flow cytometry.[9]

NEUTROPHIL BACTERIAL KILLING ASSAY

Neutrophils use both oxidative and nonoxidative mechanisms to kill microorganisms. The major steps are phagocytosis and generation of an oxidative burst. The ability of phagocytes to perform their function can be determined with a killing assay. For this test, bacteria are exposed to complement and incubated with neutrophils. The number of surviving bacteria is determined by plating the sample on an appropriate agar growth media and counting the colonies. The individual activities involved in bacterial killing can be determined using flow cytometry.

FLOW CYTOMETRY

Flow cytometry is an important tool for characterizing acquired and primary immune deficiency. Flow cytometers are used to determine characteristics of individual cells from large samples. Two physical characteristics of cells, size and granularity, are determined by the way laser light interacts with cells. This information is used by analytical flow cytometers to distinguish populations of cells into sets such as erythrocytes, lymphocytes, monocytes, and granulocytes. Antibodies and other probes, tagged with fluorescent markers, can be used to enumerate populations and subpopulations of cells. For example, the number of CD4 antigen-positive (CD4+) helper T-cell lymphocytes can be determined in a population of leukocytes based upon the binding of fluorescein tagged anti-CD4 antibody bound to the cells. Computer analysis adds an important capability to flow cytometry. The forward scatter and side scatter information used to identify lymphocytes can be combined with antibody binding information to, for example, determine not only the number of CD4+ cells in blood but the proportion of CD4+ cells within the population of lymphocytes.

Standardized cell processing procedures and gating techniques have been suggested for use in veterinary medicine.[10,11] However, there are no universally accepted procedures and different instruments, software, cell processing procedures, methods for establishing gates, and reagents hamper comparisons of data between laboratories.

REFERENCES

1. Powell AM, Leon MA. Reversible interaction of human lymphocytes with the mitogen concanavalin A. Exp Cell Res 1970;62:315–25.
2. Lyons AB. Analysing cell division in vivo and in vitro using flow cytometric measurement of CFSE dye dilution. J Immunol Methods 2000;243:147–54.
3. Mosmann T. Rapid colorimetric assay for cellular growth and survival: application to proliferation and cytotoxicity assays. J Immunol Methods 1983;65:55–63.
4. Im Hof M, Williamson L, Summerfield A, et al. Effect of synthetic agonists of toll-like receptor 9 on canine lymphocyte proliferation and cytokine production in vitro. Vet Immunol Immunopathol 2008;124:120–31.
5. Kakkis ED, Schuchman E, He X, et al. Enzyme replacement therapy in feline mucopolysaccharidosis I. Mol Genet Metab 2001;72:199–208.
6. Shull RM, Kakkis ED, McEntee MF, et al. Enzyme replacement in a canine model of Hurler syndrome. Proc Natl Acad Sci U S A 1994;91:12937–41.
7. Warman SM, Murray JK, Ridyard A, et al. Pattern of Coombs' test reactivity has diagnostic significance in dogs with immune-mediated haemolytic anaemia. J Small Anim Pract 2008;49:525–30.
8. Reimer ME, Troy GC, Warnick LD. Immune-mediated hemolytic anemia: 70 cases (1988–1996). J Am Anim Hosp Assoc 1999;35:384–91.

9. Wilkerson MJ, Davis E, Shuman W, et al. Isotype-specific antibodies in horses and dogs with immune-mediated hemolytic anemia. J Vet Intern Med 2000;14:190–6.

10. Byrne KM, Reinhart GA, Hayek MG. Standardized flow cytometry gating in veterinary medicine. Methods Cell Sci 2000;22:191–8.

11. Byrne KM, Kim HW, Chew BP, et al. A standardized gating technique for the generation of flow cytometry data for normal canine and normal feline blood lymphocytes. Vet Immunol Immunopathol 2000;73:167–82.

Immunomodulators, Immunostimulants, and Immunotherapies in Small Animal Veterinary Medicine

Eileen L. Thacker, DVM, PhD

KEYWORDS

• Small animals • Immunomodulators • Immunotherapies
• Immune system

Immunomodulators, immunostimulants and immunotherapies are important tools used by practitioners and researchers to direct and control the immune system and its response. This is a rapidly evolving field with new agents introduced, clinical trials performed, and products approved on a constant basis. Several pharmaceuticals are being tested for human use that may be useful in veterinary medicine; however, they will require further testing before they can be safely used in animals. In addition, a number of natural or herbal compounds have been reported to impact the immune system; however, frequently the scientific data to support claims is not available.

The most common use of immunomodulating agents is in downregulating the harmful immune responses that occur in autoimmune diseases and allergies. Although preventing these diseases is much easier than treating well-established, unwanted immune responses, often that is not an option. The origin of our current conventional treatments for immunologic disorders is based on screening large numbers of natural and synthetic compounds and evaluating their impact on the immune system. Conventional immune-altering drugs consist of the powerful antiinflammatory drugs of the steroid or nonsteroid group and cytotoxic drugs. Many of these compounds are derived from bacteria or fungi. These agents can be broad in their actions and inhibit the protective actions of the immune system in addition to the harmful effects. Opportunistic infections are a common consequence of the use of many of the immunosuppressive drugs.

Information on all possible products that alter the immune system cannot be covered in a single article. The goal of this article is to provide summary information on the types of the most commonly used drugs that modulate the immune system

United States Department of Agriculture - Agricultural Research Service, 5601 Sunnyside Avenue, Room 4-2104, Beltsville, MD 20705-5148, USA
E-mail address: Eileen.thacker@ars.usda.gov

Vet Clin Small Anim 40 (2010) 473–483
doi:10.1016/j.cvsm.2010.01.004   vetsmall.theclinics.com
0195-5616/10/$ – see front matter. Published by Elsevier Inc.

with examples of the most frequently used therapeutic agents within each category. In recent years, new strategies targeting specific components of the immune system have been designed. These technologies have the potential of avoiding the general suppression of the immune response observed with many of our current conventional agents; however, even these newer drugs have side effects because they affect important cells of the immune system. Examples of these experimental therapies include compounds that neutralize local cytokine and chemokine excess, target specific cell types, or manipulate the immune response to induce a more productive regulatory response. The potential for modulating the immune system of small animals through the use of immunotherapeutic strategies is great. Development of new biotechnological techniques that capitalize on our increasing information of the immune system and disease pathogenesis at the molecular and cellular level and reduce the overwhelming immune suppression of many current conventional drugs is exciting.

This article provides information on the traditional approaches to immunomodulation and stimulation, and provides information on some of the new approaches using biotechnology and more natural agents. The agents used for modulating the immune system in the treatment of inflammation, immune-mediated diseases, and neoplasms are discussed. Although one of the most important immune modulating agents is vaccines and adjuvants, they are not discussed in this article; instead the author concentrates on pharmaceutical agents used in veterinary medicine.

STEROIDAL AND NONSTEROIDAL DRUGS

Corticosteroids, pharmacologic derivatives of glucocorticoids, are used widely in veterinary medicine as antiinflammatory and immunosuppressive agents to treat autoimmune or allergic responses. These drugs have a wide range of potency and are used either alone or in combination with other immunosuppressive drugs. The long-term use of corticosteroids commonly results in side effects, including iatrogenic hyperadrenocorticism and in the event of sudden withdrawal, adrenal insufficiency. The risk for causing these side effects can be reduced by administering tailored doses so that the lowest possible level of drug is administered; by using alternate day therapy; and by using corticosteroids with intermediate duration of action, an example of which is prednisolone. Despite the risk for side effects, long-term therapy with corticosteroids may be required to prevent reoccurrence of disease. Cats are less sensitive to the immunosuppressive effects of corticosteroids and often require higher doses to alleviate disease.

Corticosteroids, such as cortisol, act through intracellular receptors of the steroid receptor superfamily and through poorly characterized membrane-bound receptors that are expressed on almost every cell of the body. After binding, the intracellular receptors bind directly to sites on the cellular DNA and either alter transcription or interact with other transcription factors, such as NFκB. In addition, corticosteroids can induce rapid production of antiinflammatory proteins by acting directly on cellular processes.[1] Corticosteroids impact a wide population of cells, are considered antiinflammatory and immunosuppressive, and may either induce or suppress as many as 20% of the genes expressed in leukocytes.[2] Given the large number of genes impacted by corticosteroids, many of which are regulated in different tissues, the effect of steroid therapy is complex. Corticosteroids regulate the expression of many genes associated with reducing inflammation. Reducing interleukin (IL) -10, tumor necrosis factor (TNF)-α, granulocyte monocyte colony stimulating factor (GM-CSF), IL-3, IL-4, IL-5, and CXCL8 are all antiinflammatory actions associated with corticosteroids.[3] Some of the other actions attributed to corticosteroids include decreased phagocytosis, antigen presentation, IL-1 production by macrophages, inhibition of complement pathways, and development of immune complexes. Additionally, corticosteroids reduce the extravasation of white cells, including margination and migration of neutrophils.[4] In dogs, prednisone increases the chemotactic responses and phagocytic activity of neutrophils.[5] Corticosteroids also reduce the number of CD4 T cells and decrease T-cell cytokines.

The various glucocorticoids have a range of potency with prednisone/prednisolone being four times and dexamethasone 30 times as potent as hydrocortisone. Thus, depending on the need, the drug used will vary depending on potency and duration needs. The prescribed uses for glucocorticoids in small animals are extensive. These drugs are commonly prescribed for treatment of several autoimmune diseases, especially atopy, although some of the newer immunosuppressive agents have been found to be more effective.[6] Glucocorticoids are some of the most commonly prescribed medicines in veterinary medicine to suppress the immune system.

In the attempt to reduce the side effects of glucocorticoids, nonsteroidal antiinflammatory drugs (NSAIDs) have been produced. The scope of these compounds on the immune system is not as dramatic, and therefore, they are not typically used for immunosuppression, as with the corticosteroids, but primarily as antiinflammatory agents. Occasionally, NSAIDs are combined with steroids, however, this is usually contraindicated because of the potentially severe side effects, including gastric ulcers and perforation.[7] Most commonly, NSAIDs are used for the management of pain associated with inflammatory joint disease and osteoarthritis.[8] The mode of action of the NSAIDs is attributed to the prevention of prostaglandin synthesis from arachidonic acid through the inhibition of cyclooxygenase (COX).[9] There are two isoenzymes of COX: COX-1, which is expressed ubiquitously in many tissues; and COX-2, which is induced by cytokines in inflamed tissues.[10] Recently, NSAIDs have been developed that specifically inhibit COX-2.[11] In addition to reducing the discomfort and inflammation, some of these agents appear to have anti-cancer abilities related to the overexpression of COX-2 by several malignancies.[12] However, more research needs to be performed to confirm this activity. Although there are several NSAIDs available for use in dogs, care must be taken in using them with cats because they are often toxic. Examples of NSAIDs include aspirin, carprofen, phenylbutazone, and flunixin meglumine. The primary side effects of NSAIDs are irritation of the gastrointestinal tract and renal problems.

T-CELL INHIBITORS

Cyclosporine A (CsA) and tacrolimus (previously known as FK506) are two immunosuppressive drugs derived from fungal and bacterial products, respectively. Originally these drugs were used to prevent organ rejection in transplant recipients. These immunosuppressant drugs are now also commonly used to treat several immune mediated diseases in dogs and cats. CsA is a cyclic decapeptide derived from *Tolypocladium inflatum*, a soil fungus in Norway. Tacrolimus is a macrolide from *Streptomyces tsukubaensis*, a filamentous bacteria found in Japan that is currently used on an experimental basis in dogs and cats. Both of these compounds bind to members of the intracellular protein family, immunophilins, and form complexes that interfere with signaling pathways in lymphocytes. CsA and tacrolimus bind to different groups of immunophilins; CsA binds to the cyclophilins and tacrolimus to the FK-binding proteins.[13]

CsA and tacrolimus block T-cell proliferation by inhibiting the phosphatase activity of calcineurin, a Ca^{2+}-activated enzyme.[13] Calcineurin is activated in T cells when intracellular calcium ion levels increase following binding of the T-cell receptor.

Upon activation, calcineurin dephosphorylates the nuclear factor of activate T-cells family of transcription factors allowing them to migrate to the nucleus where they form partners with transcription factors, such as AP-1, resulting in the transcription of genes including IL-2, CD40 ligand, and Fas ligand.[14] Tacrolimus and CsA inhibit this pathway resulting in inhibition of T-cell clonal expansion. Calcineurin is present in other cell types, but at higher levels. T cells are particularly susceptible to these drugs because of their lower levels of calcineurin.

Although originally used to prevent organ rejection following transplantation, CsA is used in veterinary medicine for the treatment of several immune-mediated diseases and allergies in dogs and cats. It has become one of the drugs of choice in the treatment of atopy in dogs and cats, being as effective as the corticosteroids with fewer side effects.[15–17] The therapeutic activity of CsA is the result of the inhibition of the inflammatory process present in allergic reactions. In addition to inhibiting T-cell activation, CsA reduces eosinophil recruitment to the sites of allergic inflammation; lymphocyte-activating functions of antigen-presenting cells, including Langerhans cells; and cytokine secretion by keratinocytes. In addition, CsA inhibits IgE and mast cell-dependent cellular infiltration.[18]

An additional use of CsA is in the treatment of keratoconjunctivitis sicca (KCS), an autoimmune disease of the lacrimal glands.[13] Administration of CsA is used in the treatment of several autoimmune diseases, including perianal fistulas, atopic dermatitis, immune-mediated hemolytic anemia, feline asthma, and the topical treatment of discoid lupus erythematosus.[19]

The most common side effects of CsA are on the gastrointestinal tract and consist of vomiting, anorexia, and diarrhea, alone or in combination.[17,20] Not all dogs are affected and side effects frequently disappear after approximately 1 week of treatment. CsA is metabolized by the liver and care must be taken in administering it to animals with hepatic disease. Other side effects reported for CsA include: heavy callusing on the footpads, red/swollen ear flaps, and proliferation of the gums. When cyclosporine is discontinued, side effects are either resolved or improved. Vaccine efficacy may be impacted by patients on CsA and the use of modified live vaccines is not recommended because of potential reactivation of the pathogen.

The primary use of tacrolimus in veterinary medicine is for the treatment of KCS.[21] Tacrolimus and CsA are the two drugs most commonly used in treating KCS. Although CsA has been the standard drug used to treat KCS, topical ophthalmic tacrolimus is considered more effective and may be useful in animals refractive to CsA treatment. Topical tacrolimus has also been used successfully in the treatment of atopic dermatitis, pemphigus, lupus erythematosus complex, military dermatitis, and the eosinophilic granuloma complex. Tacrolimus topically is well tolerated with few side effects, although gastrointestinal upset may occur when topical preparations are ingested.

New improved strategies and products to suppress the immune system will continue to be developed or adapted from human pharmaceuticals. In addition, new uses will be identified for these agents to further control inappropriate immune responses and diseases. Recently, a study showed that CsA and tacrolimus were able to inhibit replication of feline immunodeficiency virus in vitro by protecting the cells against apoptosis.[22] The results of studies such as this indicate there is the potential for increased strategies using immunosuppressive drugs for disease control in small animals.

CYTOTOXIC DRUGS

Cytotoxic drugs were originally developed to treat cancer and are now also used as immune suppressants to treat several autoimmune diseases. Two agents commonly used as immune suppressants in small animal veterinary medicine are cyclophosphamide and azathioprine. The mechanism of action of these cytotoxic drugs is through interference with DNA synthesis, acting primarily on rapidly dividing cells.[18] Cyclophosphamide is an alkylating agent, causing breakage or cross linking between or within DNA strands. This action interferes with DNA replication and RNA transcription and as a result impacts dividing and intermitotic cells, thus being cell-cycle nonspecific. Cyclophosphamide is a member of the nitrogen mustard family that was originally developed as chemical weapons.

The thiopurines, of which azathioprine is an example, act on the S phase of the cell cycle, competing with adenine and substituting nonsense bases during nucleic acid synthesis. Studies have suggested that azathioprine may have a preferential suppressive effect on T-cell immunity.[23] Azathioprine also interferes with CD28 co-stimulation, leading to the generation of an apoptotic signal through the blockade of the small GTPase Rac1, a small G-protein of the Rho family.[18]

The use of these drugs results in several toxic effects on tissues with dividing cells, such as skin, gut lining, and bone marrow. Effects include decreased immune function, anemia, leucopenia, thrombocytopenia, and damage to intestinal epithelium. These drugs are used in high doses to eliminate all dividing lymphocytes as would be the case of preliminary treatment to a bone marrow transplant. Lower levels are used either alone or in combination to treat either neoplasias or unwanted immune responses.

Cyclophosphamide is used in dogs and cats as a part of the multidrug induction protocol in the treatment of lymphoma. Cyclophosphamide is frequently combined with several other chemotherapeutic agents, including vincristine.[24] Cyclophosphamide has been used to treat several immune-mediated diseases, including glomerulonephritis, feline infectious peritonitis, polyarthritis, and chronic inflammatory polyneuropathy. Cyclophosphamide is no longer used in the treatment of immune-mediated, autoimmune hemolytic anemia because prednisone alone has increased efficacy and cyclophosphamide does not resolve the hemolysis more rapidly.[25,26]

A side effect of cyclophosphamide is myelosuppression, which can have a dose-limiting effect. Within 5 to 14 days, neutropenia may occur, which may take as long as 4 weeks to resolve after the drug is discontinued. In contrast, thrombocytopenia rarely occurs. Gastrointestinal side effects, including vomiting, diarrhea, and anorexia, may occur. Anorexia is more frequent in cats. Bladder toxicity may occur in dogs and cats because of the effect of the metabolite acrolein on the bladder urothelium, and may result in sterile-hemorrhagic cystitis. Coadministration of furosemide has been reported to decrease the incidence of cyclophosphamide-induced cystitis (http://www.wedgewoodpharmacy.com/monographs/cyclophosphamide.asp).

Azathioprine is used in the treatment of a number of immune-mediated disorders including inflammatory bowel disease; immune-mediated anemia, colitis, and skin disease; and Myasthenia Gravis. Azathioprine is commonly combined with prednisone or other corticosteroid to reduce the dose of both drugs and allow alternate day use. The onset of action of azathioprine is delayed, taking between 3 and 6 weeks to occur.

The incidence of myelosuppression associated with azathioprine therapy is controlled by the level of thioprine methyltransferase (TMPT), an enzyme involved in azathioprine metabolism.[23] Cats are susceptible to azathioprine toxicity because they have low levels of TMPT. The TMPT activity in dogs and myelosuppression is more variable.

As with cyclophosphamide, gastrointestinal side effects are common with azathioprine. In addition, pancreatitis and reduced liver function may occur and liver function tests are recommended before use. Concurrent administration of glucocorticoids, which is fairly common, increases the risk for toxicity. (http://www.wedgewoodpharmacy.com/monographs/azathioprine.asp).

IMMUNOSTIMULATORS AND BIOLOGIC RESPONSE MODIFIERS

Products that stimulate the immune response in a nonspecific manner are used widely as immunostimulators. The most common immunostimulators used in veterinary medicine are the adjuvants that are added to vaccines to stimulate an immune response to the antigen. As our knowledge of the immune system increases, these products are becoming more refined to enable specific arms or cells of the immune system to be stimulated. In addition, the exact type of immune response needed to produce an enhanced immune response, whether it is to a vaccine, in response to disease, or even to prevent disease, can be accomplished with several specific agents. Adjuvants are not discussed in this article; however, their role in vaccinology is as immunostimulators.

Several additional immunomodulating agents are used in dogs and cats for treating a variety of immune-mediated disorders. An example of a unique immunomodulator is Lymphocyte T-Cell Immune Modulator (LTCI) (IMULAN BioTherapeutics, LLC St. Joseph, MO). The mode of action of LTCI is through the regulation of CD-4+ T lymphocytes.[27] Use of LTCI has been shown to increase the number of lymphocytes and IL-2. The active ingredient of LTCI is a 50,000 dalton protein isolated from cloned thymic epithelial cells. CD-4+ lymphocytes are important mediators of immunity and are often adversely impacted by viral infections resulting in decreased numbers or function of CD-4+ lymphocytes. Viral infections often result in the production of IL-2 and interferon gamma is reduced, both of which are produced by CD4+ cells and are required to activate CD8+ lymphocytes, which are important in the destruction and control of virally infected cells.[28] In addition to increasing the number and activity of CD4+ lymphocytes, LTCI promotes hematopoiesis, including red blood cells, platelets, and granulocytes. By impacting CD4+ lymphocytes, LTCI enhances the immune response to viruses. Biochemically, LTCI is a single chain polypeptide. Produced from bovine-derived stromal cell supernatant, it is a strongly cationic glycoprotein. It is approved as an aid in the treatment of cats infected with feline leukemia virus (FeLV) or feline immunodeficiency virus (FIV) and their associated blood disorders.[27]

Levamisole, which is primarily used in veterinary medicine as an anthelminthic in production animals, has also been described as an immunostimulant and as a vaccine adjuvant that enhances the activity of T and B lymphocytes in dogs.[29] Activation of T lymphocytes and increased antibody production has been reported when levamisole is used as an adjuvant. Increased function of monocytes and neutrophils has been reported, as well as enhancing maturation of dendritic cells. In addition, upregulation and expression of toll-like receptor (TLR) 7 and 8 and MyD99 occur. Downregulation of suppression signaling of the Janus kinases/signal transducers and activators of transcription (JAK/STAT) pathway has been reported.[29] Thus, activation of the innate immune system while downregulating suppression mechanisms may enhance the immune response. The mode of action is through effecting the metabolism of cyclic nucleotides (S-AMP, c-GMP). The use of levamisole has been reported to produce long-term remission in more than 50% of dogs with systemic lupus erythematosus when administered in combination with prednisolone.[19] In this therapeutic regimen, the prednisolone dose is decreased over 1 to 2 months and discontinued, whereas levamisole is administered continuously for 4 months and then stopped. Recurrence of disease is treated with levamisole alone for an additional 4 months.

HERBAL IMMUNE MODULATORS

There are several herbs or extracts that have been reported to impact the immune system. Some of the claims have scientific merit, whereas others have only anecdotal support. Verifying claims for many of these compounds can be challenging because growing and extracting procedures can alter the active ingredient level and activity resulting in variation within and between products. As a result, care must be taken to ensure that the products are safe in the species of interest and that dosing might differ between levels reported in the literature and the various products used.

Some plants known as adaptogens have been shown in clinical trials to increase resistance to stress, thus increasing resistance to disease.[30] These herbs generally work through modulation of the hypothalamic-pituitary-adrenal axis, but other mechanisms may also be involved with immune modulation. The best known plant in this group is Asian Ginseng (*Panax ginseng*). Stress models in rats found that pretreatment with ginseng attenuated the stress-induced rise in corticosteroids and immune suppression. Other examples of adaptogens reported to impact the immune system include American ginseng (*Panax quinquefolius*), Eleuthero (*Eleutherococcus senticosis*), and Ashwagandha (*Withania somnifera*).[30]

Other natural products work as immune modulators; however, the efficacy of many of these herbs is poorly documented or studies have been conducted in vitro or on laboratory animals and not necessarily the species of interest. Immune stimulating herbs have been observed to reactivate or increase the severity of autoimmune diseases, so care must be taken when prescribing them to patients. Examples of these types of immune stimulators include various medicinal fungi, such as Shitake (*Lentinula edodes*) or Reishi (*Ganoderma lucidum*), which contain polysaccharide complexes and sterols.[30] These fungi have been attributed with enhancing cell mediated immunity and may have antitumor activities. Echinacea (*Echinacea* spp) is one of the more recognized herbs associated with immune modulation. In humans, it has been reported to impact the innate immune system by increasing the activity of phagocytic cells, promoting production of various cytokines, and enhancing the activity of natural killer cells.[31] Little work has been done in small animals, although studies in swine and horses suggest that the immune modulating activities can occur in domestic animals. Long-term use of Echinacea has been associated with toxicity or autoimmunity, although this has not been documented.[32] There are several other herbs reported to modulate the immune system including Astragalus (*Astragalus membranaceus*), which is reported to increase T-cell mediated immunity; Ginseng polysaccharides; and saponins. The claims of these agents have been in laboratory rodents and uncontrolled human trials, so care must be taken in their use.[30]

Other natural immune modulators include the CpG oligodeoxynucleotides (CpG ODN) from specific bacterial DNA nucleotide sequences. These sequences, which are underrepresented in vertebrate genomes and when present are methylated, are thought to be recognized as foreign resulting in an immune response. The CpG ODNs induce a systemic innate immune response of short duration that occurs quickly after exposure. Studies have demonstrated that CpG ODNs stimulate B-cell proliferation, expression, and production of cytokines and enhanced NK cell cytotoxicity.[33] CpG ODN sequences induce lymphocyte proliferation of canine and feline spleen and lymph node cells.[34] This technology is promising for use as vaccine adjuvants, immunotherapy for cancer, and to redirect inappropriate T helper 2 allergic immune responses toward a T helper 1 immune response.[35,36]

More directed use of immunostimulants includes the use of Staphylococcus Aureus Phage Lysate (Staphage Lysate or SPL, Delmont Laboratories, Inc, Swarthmore, PA, USA), which has been used in treatment of canine pyoderma caused by staphylococcal hypersensitivity.[37] This preparation contains a bacteriophage and has been demonstrated to increase the capability of macrophages to inactivate staphylococci.

Other more natural treatments for immunity against pathogens or autoimmune diseases include cytokines or chemokines. The advent of creating and administering specific cytokines allows the fine tuning and directing of immune responses down a specific pathway, which ensures that the immune response generated is tailored to the need, whether it is to a pathogen, an autoimmune disorder, neoplasia, or nonspecific prevention of disease. To date, cytokines have been used in dogs and cats primarily to treat viral diseases and to induce enhanced immunity against tumors. In dogs, interferon-omega has been used successfully to treat canine parvovirus infections.[38,39] In cats, several immunomodulating agents have been used to treat FeLV and FIV infections with varied success.[40] In addition, a study reported using liposome-IL2 DNA complex to stimulate the immune system in cats with chronic rhinitis.[41] Only adult cats showed any response, but these types of novel therapies provide new opportunities to explore and develop intervention strategies for diseases that have proved problematic in the past.

NEOPLASIA CHEMOTHERAPEUTIC AGENTS

Several chemotherapeutic agents act against neoplasias through immunomodulatory action. The theory behind using immunostimulants/immunomodulatory agents for treatment of neoplasias is to activate the immune system to recognize the tumor as foreign and destroy it. Many of these agents are nonspecific immune modulators. Many of the agents currently used to treat autoimmune disorders, such as cyclophosphamide, that were discussed earlier in this article were originally used to treat various neoplasias. In addition, studies have found that agents, such as NSAIDs and levamisole, may also have anti-cancer activities. It is not within the scope of this article to discuss all chemotherapeutic agents used to treat cancer.

An example of an immunostimulating agent used to treat canine and feline neoplasms includes the polysaccharide acemannan. Acemannan Immunostimulant consists of long-chain polydispersed β-(1,4)-linked mannan polymers interspersed with O-acetyl groups and is extracted from aloe vera (*barbadensis Miller*).[42] The mechanism of action of Acemannan is thought to be through macrophage activation and release of TNF, IL-1, and interferon. Use of Acemannan has been reported to have resulted in significant changes in tumors of 26 out of 43 dogs and cats.[43] The histopathologic results found in the 26 cases included marked necrosis or lymphocytic infiltration of the tumors. Thirteen of the animals showed moderate to marked tumor necrosis or liquefaction. Twelve animals had clinical improvement as determined by reduced tumor size, tumor necrosis, or prolonged survival. Five of seven animals with fibrosarcomas had positive results. With repeated injections, systemic toxicity was limited, with accumulation of macrophages and monocytes in either the lungs or liver and spleen depending on location of injection. The effects were not considered adverse, but were consistent with the immune stimulating activity of Acemannan.[44]

Other examples of immune stimulating or modulating nonspecific agents include the use of IL-2, interferon gamma (IFN-γ), IL-12, GM-CSF, or CD40L.[45,46] Use of many of these agents has resulted in reduced size or regression of tumors and prolonged life of the animal treated. Depending on the type of cancer, size, and prognosis, the use of these immunostimulating cytokines show great potential in veterinary medicine for the treatment of tumors. More specific therapies using tumor antigens, monoclonal antibodies, and cancer vaccines are also available. Many of these types of individualized therapies are expensive as specific antigens of the neoplasias need to be isolated and use as the target for these vaccines. This requires collaboration with specialized laboratories and is not currently routinely available. Frequently, the cytokines described earlier are included to enhance the immunogenicity of the tumor antigens. These therapies allow the animals' own immune system to destroy the tumor, often resulting in significantly fewer side effects than with cytotoxic drugs or radiation.

SUMMARY

The objective of this article is to provide a summary and overview of some of the potential immunomodulatory and immunostimulating agents currently being investigated or used in companion animals. Some of the agents described are currently approved for use, whereas others are either in preliminary research phases or reportedly used in other species. It is important to recognize that therapy that impacts the immune system, whether in a positive or negative fashion, is a rapidly growing area of research and as our knowledge of the immune system of domestic animals increases, new opportunities and pharmaceutical agents will be developed. As stated earlier, the ultimate immunomodulatory agents are vaccines, which stimulate the immune system to prevent disease, or even neoplasias and are not discussed in this article. However, as with the currently available pharmaceutical agents, novel adjuvants will be developed to further enhance the immune response to antigens as we begin to understand the immune system at the cellular and molecular levels.

REFERENCES

1. Kampa M, Castanas E. Membrane steroid receptor signaling in normal and neoplastic cells. Mol Cell Endocrinol 2006;246:76.
2. Galon J, Franchimont D, Hiroi N, et al. Gene profiling reveals unknown enhancing and suppressive actions of glucocorticoids on immune cells. FASEB J 2002;16:61.
3. Rhen T, Cidlowski JA. Antiinflammatory action of glucocorticoids–new mechanisms for old drugs. N Engl J Med 2005;353:1711.
4. Dannenberg AM Jr. The antiinflammatory effects of glucocorticosteroids. A brief review of the literature. Inflammation 1979;3:329.
5. Rinkardt NE, Kruth SA, Kaushik A. The effects of prednisone and azathioprine on circulating immunoglobulin levels and lymphocyte subpopulations in normal dogs. Can J Vet Res 1999;63:18.
6. Olivry T, Mueller RS. Evidence-based veterinary dermatology: a systematic review of the pharmacotherapy of canine atopic dermatitis. Vet Dermatol 2003;14:121.
7. Mathews KA. Nonsteroidal anti-inflammatory analgesics in pain management in dogs and cats. Can Vet J 1996;37:539.
8. Sanderson RO, Beata C, Flipo RM, et al. Systematic review of the management of canine osteoarthritis. Vet Rec 2009;164:418.
9. Clark TP. The clinical pharmacology of cyclooxygenase-2-selective and dual inhibitors. Vet Clin North Am Small Anim Pract 2006;36:1061.
10. Narita T, Sato R, Motoishi K, et al. The interaction between orally administered non-steroidal anti-inflammatory drugs and prednisolone in healthy dogs. J Vet Med Sci 2007;69:353.
11. Streppa HK, Jones CJ, Budsberg SC. Cyclooxygenase selectivity of nonsteroidal anti-inflammatory drugs in canine blood. Am J Vet Res 2002;63:91.
12. Boonsoda S, Wanikiat P. Possible role of cyclooxygenase-2 inhibitors as anti-cancer agents. Vet Rec 2008;162:159.
13. Moore CP. Immunomodulating agents. Vet Clin North Am Small Anim Pract 2004; 34:725.
14. Bierer BE, Mattila PS, Standaert RF, et al. Two distinct signal transmission pathways in T lymphocytes are inhibited by complexes formed between an

immunophilin and either FK506 or rapamycin. Proc Natl Acad Sci U S A 1990; 87:9231.

15. Steffan J, Favrot C, Mueller R. A systematic review and meta-analysis of the efficacy and safety of cyclosporin for the treatment of atopic dermatitis in dogs. Vet Dermatol 2006;17:3.

16. Steffan J, Strehlau G, Maurer M, et al. Cyclosporin A pharmacokinetics and efficacy in the treatment of atopic dermatitis in dogs. J Vet Pharmacol Ther 2004;27:231.

17. Wisselink MA, Willemse T. The efficacy of cyclosporine A in cats with presumed atopic dermatitis: a double blind, randomised prednisolone-controlled study. Vet J 2009;180:55.

18. Murphy K, Travers P, Walport M. Janeway's Immunobiology. New York: Garland Science, Taylor & Francis Group, LLC; 2008.

19. Day MJ. Clinical immunology of the dog and cat. Ames (IA): Iowa State University Press; 1999.

20. Radowicz SN, Power HT. Long-term use of cyclosporine in the treatment of canine atopic dermatitis. Vet Dermatol 2005;16:81.

21. Moore CP. Ocular therapeutics. Vet Clin North Am Small Anim Pract 2004;34:XI.

22. Mortola E, Endo Y, Ohno K, et al. The use of two immunosuppressive drugs, cyclosporin A and tacrolimus, to inhibit virus replication and apoptosis in cells infected with feline immunodeficiency virus. Vet Res Commun 1998;22:553.

23. Rodriguez DB, Mackin A, Easley R, et al. Relationship between red blood cell thiopurine methyltransferase activity and myelotoxicity in dogs receiving azathioprine. J Vet Intern Med 2004;18:339.

24. Cave TA, Norman P, Mellor D. Cytotoxic drug use in treatment of dogs and cats with cancer by UK veterinary practices (2003 to 2004). J Small Anim Pract 2007; 48:371.

25. Goggs R, Boag AK, Chan DL. Concurrent immune-mediated haemolytic anaemia and severe thrombocytopenia in 21 dogs. Vet Rec 2008;163:323.

26. Piek CJ, Junius G, Dekker A, et al. Idiopathic immune-mediated hemolytic anemia: treatment outcome and prognostic factors in 149 dogs. J Vet Intern Med 2008;22:366.

27. Gingerich DA. Lymphocyte T-Cell immunomodulator (LTCI): review of the immunopharmacology of a new veterinary biologic. J Appl Res Vet Med 2008;6:61.

28. de Mari K, Maynard L, Sanquer A, et al. Therapeutic effects of recombinant feline interferon-omega on feline leukemia virus (FeLV)-infected and FeLV/feline immunodeficiency virus (FIV)-coinfected symptomatic cats. J Vet Intern Med 2004;18: 477.

29. Zhang W, Du X, Zhao G, et al. Levamisole is a potential facilitator for the activation of Th1 responses of the subunit HBV vaccination. Vaccine 2009;27:4938.

30. Wynn SG, Fougere B. Veterinary herbal medicine: a systems-based approach. In: Wynn SG, Fougere B, editors. Veterinary herbal medicine. New York: Mosby/ Elsevier; 2007. p. 291.

31. Sullivan AM, Laba JG, Moore JA, et al. Echinacea-induced macrophage activation. Immunopharmacol Immunotoxicol 2008;30:553.

32. Gryzlak BM, Wallace RB, Zimmerman MB, et al. National surveillance of herbal dietary supplement exposures: the poison control center experience. Pharmacoepidemiol Drug Saf 2007;16:947.

33. Klaschik S, Tross D, Shirota H, et al. Short- and long-term changes in gene expression mediated by the activation of TLR9. Mol Immunol, December 17, 2009. [Online].

34. Wernette CM, Smith BF, Barksdale ZL, et al. CpG oligodeoxynucleotides stimulate canine and feline immune cell proliferation. Vet Immunol Immunopathol 2002;84:223.
35. Hayashi M, Satou E, Ueki R, et al. Resistance to influenza A virus infection by antigen-conjugated CpG oligonucleotides, a novel antigen-specific immunomodulator. Biochem Biophys Res Commun 2005;329:230.
36. Reinero CR, Cohn LA, Delgado C, et al. Adjuvanted rush immunotherapy using CpG oligodeoxynucleotides in experimental feline allergic asthma. Vet Immunol Immunopathol 2008;121:241.
37. DeBoer DJ, Moriello KA, Thomas CB, et al. Evaluation of a commercial staphylococcal bacteria for management of idiopathic recurrent superficial pyoderma in dogs. Am J Vet Res 1990;51:636.
38. de Mari K, Maynard L, Eun HM, et al. Treatment of canine parvoviral enteritis with interferon-omega in a placebo-controlled field trial. Vet Rec 2003;152:105.
39. Kuwabara M, Nariai Y, Horiuchi Y, et al. Immunological effects of recombinant feline interferon-omega (KT-80) administration in the dog. Microbiol Immunol 2006;50:637.
40. Nagashima N, Hisasue M, Nishigaki K, et al. In vitro selective suppression of feline myeloid colony formation is attributable to molecularly cloned strain of feline leukemia virus with unique long terminal repeat. Res Vet Sci 2005;78:151.
41. Veir JK, Lappin MR, Dow SW. Evaluation of a novel immunotherapy for treatment of chronic rhinitis in cats. J Feline Med Surg 2006;8:400.
42. Talmadge J, Chavez J, Jacobs L, et al. Fractionation of Aloe vera L. inner gel, purification and molecular profiling of activity. Int Immunopharmacol 2004;4:1757.
43. Harris C, Pierce K, King G, et al. Efficacy of acemannan in treatment of canine and feline spontaneous neoplasms. Mol Biother 1991;3:207.
44. Fogleman RW, Chapdelaine JM, Carpenter RH, et al. Toxicologic evaluation of injectable acemannan in the mouse, rat and dog. Vet Hum Toxicol 1992;34:201.
45. Jahnke A, Hirschberger J, Fischer C, et al. Intra-tumoral gene delivery of feIL-2, feIFN-gamma and feGM-CSF using magnetofection as a neoadjuvant treatment option for feline fibrosarcomas: a phase-I study. J Vet Med A Physiol Pathol Clin Med 2007;54:599.
46. von Euler H, Sadeghi A, Carlsson B, et al. Efficient adenovector CD40 ligand immunotherapy of canine malignant melanoma. J Immunother 2008;31:377.

Transfusion Medicine in Small Animal Practice

Lynel J. Tocci, DVM, MT(ASCP)SBB

KEYWORDS

- Hemagglutination • Blood typing • Crossmatching
- Blood transfusion • Transfusion reaction

Red blood cell (RBC) transfusions in veterinary medicine have become increasingly more common and are an integral part of lifesaving and advanced treatment of the critically ill. Common situations involving transfusions are life-threatening anemia from acute hemorrhage or surgical blood loss, hemolysis from drugs or toxins, immune-mediated diseases, severe nonregenerative conditions, and neonatal isoerythrolysis. A wide variety of blood types exist in domestic animals, and new antigens are being discovered with increasing frequency. Today, it is not uncommon to have patients with previous transfusion histories requiring additional transfusions, and now there are rapid and reliable point-of-care tests for blood typing and crossmatching. Pretransfusion testing is designed to help ensure that an RBC transfusion is effective while minimizing the risk of adverse reactions (immediate or delayed). Although transfusions can be lifesaving, they are also associated with adverse events that can be life threatening. This article reviews the principles for pretransfusion blood typing and compatibility testing and the types of transfusion reactions that exist despite test performance.

THE STRUCTURE OF ANTIBODIES

Immunoglobulins are the proteins that are either cell bound and serve as antigen receptors on B lymphocytes or secreted by plasma cells in soluble form as antibodies. Five general types or classes of immunoglobulin antibodies are produced, and the same basic structural component gives rise to all the immunoglobulin molecules. Each immunoglobulin is a symmetric unit containing 4 polypeptide chains, 2 long heavy chains and 2 short light chains. There are 2 types of light chains, κ and λ and 5 types of heavy chains, μ, γ, α, δ, and ε. It is the heavy chain that determines the antibody classes IgM, IgG, IgA, IgD, and IgE, respectively. IgM is the first antibody class to be synthesized and secreted into the plasma in a primary immune response and is

Department of Emergency and Critical Care, Veterinary Emergency & Specialty Center of New England, 180 Bear Hill Road, Waltham, MA 02454, USA
E-mail address: ltocci@vescone.com

Vet Clin Small Anim 40 (2010) 485–494
doi:10.1016/j.cvsm.2010.02.005
0195-5616/10/$ – see front matter © 2010 Published by Elsevier Inc.

efficient at binding complement. IgG is produced in large quantities during a secondary immune response. Red cell alloantibodies are IgM, IgG, or IgE antibodies and cause hypersensitivity reactions to blood products.[1]

The immune response is highly evolved and has the ability to distinguish self from nonself. Each antibody produced as part of this response is specific for a particular antigen. The specificity between an antibody and its corresponding antigen is a reversible reaction that obeys the thermodynamic mass action law.

$$K_0 = \frac{\text{concentration of bound antibody} - \text{antigen}}{\text{concentration of antibody} \times \text{concentration of antigen}}$$

K_0 is the affinity constant and is a measure of how tight an antibody binds with its corresponding antigen. K_0 is determined by the rate of association and dissociation of the reaction. There is an equilibrium between free antigen, free antibody, and the complex of antigen and antibody. The binding affinity or strength of the interaction is a measure of the goodness of fit.[2]

Immunohematology is the study of antigens and antibodies associated with blood transfusions and complications of pregnancy, such as neonatal isoerythrolysis. Reactions between RBC antigens and plasma antibodies can be detected in testing methods. The principle of human and veterinary blood typing and compatibility methods is a visible hemagglutination reaction. Agglutination is the endpoint for most tests involving red cells and blood group antibodies. Agglutination is the antibody-mediated clumping of cells that express antigen on their surface. It occurs in 2 stages: (1) sensitization, antibody attaching to antigen on the RBC membrane and (2) crosslinking, the formation of bridges by antibodies between sensitized red cells to form the lattice that constitutes agglutination. For sensitization to occur, antigen and antibody must come in close apposition, and for cross-linking to occur, the antibody must be able to bind with antigens on each of 2 red cells.[2] In tests for detecting antibodies to RBC antigens, hemolysis is also a positive test, as it demonstrates the agglutination of an antibody with an antigen that activates the complement cascade.

BLOOD GROUPS

Blood groups are defined by inherited antigens on the RBC surface. These genetic markers are species specific and vary in immunogenicity and clinical significance. RBC antigens contribute to the recognition of self and can elicit the production of an antibody when introduced into the circulation of an animal whose RBCs lack that antigen. This becomes significant in situations of RBC transfusions and neonatal isoerythrolysis in which hemolytic reactions can occur.

CANINE BLOOD TYPES

The 7 internationally recognized canine blood groups are categorized under the dog erythrocyte antigen (DEA) system. By convention, the canine blood types are designated using the DEA acronym, followed by the numerical designation of the blood group. DEAs 1.1, 1.2, 3, 4, 5, 6, 7, and 8 have been identified, and typing antisera is available for all, except DEA 6 and DEA 8.[3,4] Beyond the internationally recognized blood groups, a new antigen referred to as Dal has been described. This newly recognized antigen was found to have no correlation with the known DEA antigens.[5] Currently, DEAs 1.1 and 1.2 are considered important in transfusion medicine. DEA 1.1 is known to be extremely antigenic, and DEA 1.1 negative dogs exposed to DEA

1.1 positive RBCs likely become sensitized and produce an anti–DEA 1.1 alloantibody. Subsequent transfusions of DEA 1.1 positive RBC in the DEA 1.1 negative patient result in an acute hemolytic crisis. Therefore, DEA 1.1 is the antigen routinely determined in patients and donors, and 42% of the canine population is positive.[4] An acute hemolytic transfusion reaction (AHTR) has been reported in a DEA 1.1 negative dog, which had developed antibodies to DEA 1.1 from a previous transfusion of DEA 1.1 positive RBC.[6] A serious hemolytic transfusion reaction has also been reported in a previously sensitized DEA 4 negative dog from exposure to DEA 4 positive RBC.[7] Unlike DEA 1.1, the DEA 4 antigen has high prevalence, and 98% of dogs are reported to be positive. Naturally occurring alloantibodies to DEAs 3, 5, and 7 occur in dogs negative for these antigens and cause delayed RBC survival.[3,4] A corresponding antibody (anti-Dal) to the Dal antigen has also been reported. This antibody was transfusion induced in a Dal-negative patient.[5]

At this time, there is no consensus as to the universal canine donor. The ideal universal canine donor would be negative for the most common antigens other than those of high frequency (eg, DEA 4).[4] At minimum, the canine donor RBC unit should be typed for DEA 1.1 and labeled as positive or negative. Ideally, the blood typing of the recipient should also be performed. However, in emergent situations, DEA 1.1 negative RBCs can be given if the blood type is unknown. Fortunately, without prior sensitization, dogs do not possess naturally occurring alloantibodies to DEA 1.1, and if necessary, the first transfusion to a DEA 1.1 negative dog with DEA 1.1 positive RBC is unlikely to cause an immediate problem. These recipients become sensitized to the DEA 1.1 antigen and make a strong agglutinating and hemolyzing anti–DEA 1.1 alloantibody. Subsequent transfusions should be DEA 1.1 negative and crossmatch compatible. Extended blood typing beyond DEA 1.1 would be indicated with incompatible crossmatches or transfusion reactions.

FELINE BLOOD TYPES

Until recently, the feline AB blood group system was thought to be limited to 3 blood types: type A, type B, and type AB. Similar to humans, all type A and type B cats possess naturally occurring alloantibodies against the blood group antigen they lack. These alloantibodies are responsible for hemolytic transfusion reactions in mismatched or incompatible RBC transfusions and in cases of neonatal isoerytholysis.[8–11] Feline type A is the predominant type worldwide, and incidence varies with breed and geographic location. The highest frequency of type B cats has been reported in the Devon Rex and British Shorthair and in nonpurebred Australian cats.[8–10] Additional antigens outside the AB blood group have been suspected based on type-specific incompatible crossmatches. A new antigen Mik has recently been described. The investigators also report a naturally occurring alloantibody, anti-Mik, in Mik antigen negative cats.[12]

A universal feline blood donor does not exist. Blood typing should be performed in all donors and patients, and a crossmatch in addition to blood typing is recommended.

BLOOD TYPING METHODS

The principle of all veterinary blood typing methods is a visible hemagglutination reaction between patient RBC surface antigens and known reagent monoclonal or polyclonal antisera. The International Society of Animal Genetics is responsible for the standardization of blood typing reagents. The availability of blood typing reagents for extended blood typing is limited. For the dog DEA 1.1, typing is commercially available and for the cat types A, B, and AB can be determined. Commercial methods include typing cards (DMS Laboratories, Flemington, NJ, USA), gel column (DiaMed, Switzerland), and immunochromatographic cartridges (Alvedia, France).

CROSSMATCHING

Allogenic blood transfusions have the potential to introduce foreign antigens into the recipient. The major crossmatch is the serologic method designed to determine the compatibility between the donor RBC and the recipient (patient). The main purpose of the test is to help prevent incompatible transfusions that could result in immune-mediated hemolytic transfusion reactions. Donor RBCs are incubated with recipient serum and observed for visible agglutination or hemolysis. If an agglutination reaction or hemolysis occurs, an incompatibility exists and the donor RBCs should not be used for the transfusion. Causes of incompatibility occur if the recipient has a naturally occurring or an induced alloantibody directed against an antigen present on the donor RBCs. If no agglutination or hemolysis is noted, the crossmatch is considered compatible and the RBCs acceptable for transfusion.

The minor crossmatch is the serologic method designed to determine the compatibility between the donor plasma and the recipient (patient). The transfusion of plasma-containing components (whole blood, fresh frozen plasma) has the potential to cause destruction of the recipient RBCs if the donor has an alloantibody directed against an RBC antigen present on the recipient's RBCs.

Compatible major crossmatch, minor crossmatch, or both does not guarantee normal RBC survival or completely eliminate the risk of the transfusion. Delayed transfusion reactions and reactions to donor leukocytes or plasma proteins are not prevented by crossmatching.

CROSSMATCHING METHODS

In human medicine, the crossmatch was first described in 1907 and has been modified multiple times. Major milestones in its evolution include multiple rapid techniques, from test tube to gel, and multiple types of enhancement media, such as high protein, enzymes, and antiglobulin. If a slide or tube technique is used, the experience of the person performing the test is of high importance. Slide or tube agglutination reactions should be evaluated by a medical technologist or other appropriately trained individual to assure accurate interpretation. In small animal veterinary medicine, the saline agglutination or the indirect antiglobulin tube crossmatch is used. If performed correctly, these tube techniques should identify potential transfusion incompatibilities. However, the test can be time consuming and cumbersome and is most often reserved for the clinical laboratory setting. An alternative method, gel agglutination, is currently available in veterinary practice for canine and feline crossmatching. The test is less time consuming, standardized, and does not require a medical technologist for interpretation. In addition, reactions are stable and can be reviewed by multiple people at a later time. To date, there have been no published veterinary studies comparing crossmatching via tube assay with the gel agglutination method. However, the investigators of Dal antigen used a gel technology in conjunction with a standard tube technology for crossmatching and reported agreement of both methods.[5] In human medicine, the gel test is comparable with the tube assay for both the indirect and direct antiglobulin tests.[13–16] There are currently 2 commercially available gel tests for canine and feline crossmatching: DiaMed-ID (crossmatching gel; DiaMed, Switzerland) and Rapid Vet-H (companion animal crossmatch gel; DMS Laboratories,

Inc, Flemington, NJ, USA). A standardized tube crossmatch procedure is described in numerous veterinary tests.[17-19]

TRANSFUSION REACTIONS

The transfusion of any blood component presents a risk to the recipient. Adverse reactions can occur despite pretransfusion testing, and therefore, transfusion therapy requires careful analysis of the risks and benefits of the therapy by the clinician. Proper donor screening and collection as well as proper processing and storage of blood components minimize the risks of adverse reactions. Transfusion reactions are categorized as immunologic and nonimmunologic and as acute or delayed. Immunologic reactions are caused by RBCs, plasma proteins, white blood cells (WBCs) or platelet antigens or antibodies. AHTRs are the most serious and potentially life threatening, and febrile and allergic transfusion reactions make up most immediate reactions.

Acute Immunologic Transfusion Reactions

Immune-mediated hemolysis

AHTRs occur when transfused RBCs interact with preformed circulating antibodies in the recipient that are naturally occurring or acquired. The interaction of the recipient's antibody with the donor RBC antigen can activate complement and cytokines and result in a systemic inflammatory response. The severity of the response is directly related to the number of RBCs destroyed. The reactions are predominantly IgG mediated in the dog and IgM mediated in the cat.[18] Clinical signs may include fever, restlessness, salivation, incontinence, and shock. Consequences of intravascular hemolysis are hemoglobinemia, hemoglobinuria, vasoconstriction, renal ischemia and acute renal failure, disseminated intravascular coagulopathy, and death. The treatment of an AHTR depends on the severity. Treatment of hypotension and maintaining adequate renal blood flow are primary concerns. When an AHTR is suspected, stop the transfusion and begin crystalloid and/or colloid infusion to optimize blood pressure (mean 60–70 mm Hg) and maintain renal perfusion and urine output (1–2 mL/kg/h).

Febrile nonhemolytic reactions

A febrile nonhemolytic transfusion reaction (FNHTR) is often defined as a temperature increase of more than 1°C associated with a transfusion without any other explanation. These reactions are most likely associated with leukocyte-derived cytokine and/or circulating antileukocyte (WBC) antibodies in the recipient (patient). FNHTRs are associated with chills and rigors.[20,21] Most reactions are benign although some may cause hemodynamic or respiratory changes. Because fever may be the initial manifestation of an AHTR or a reaction to a bacterial contaminated unit, any observed temperature increase associated with a transfusion warrants attention. In people, FNHTRs respond to antipyretics, and acetaminophen is preferred to salicylates; antihistamines are not indicated.[22] In addition, pretreatment before transfusion is contraindicated. The use of acetaminophen in veterinary patients is contraindicated, as its toxicity is a result of N-acetyl-p-quinoneimine, an intermediate product that cannot be cleared because of the lack of adequate amounts of glutathione in veterinary patients, limiting detoxification and causing hepatic toxicity. Treating an FNHTR in small animals consists of slowing or temporarily stopping the transfusion and administering a nonsteroidal antiinflammatory drug that is safe to use in small animals.

Allergic reactions

Allergic reactions can be mild, as in the form of hives, or severe, as in the form of anaphylaxis with hypotension, shock, and in some cases, death. The term "anaphylactoid" is used to describe allergic reactions between the mild and severe extremes. IgE is the antibody that mediates type I hypersensitivity reactions and the antibody responsible for most allergic reactions. However, IgG and IgA antibodies may also induce an allergic or anaphylactic response.[21,23] IgE-mediated allergic reactions are caused by soluble substances in the donor plasma that binds to preformed IgE antibodies on mast cells in the recipient, resulting in the activation and release of histamine. Complement fixation with IgG causes the release of C3a and C5a anaphylatoxins.[22] Fever is characteristically absent in people. If hives are the only adverse event, the transfusion can be temporarily interrupted and an antihistamine (eg, diphenhydramine) administered. The transfusion can be resumed when symptoms are resolved. If hives and respiratory and/or gastrointestinal signs are present or the patient is hypotensive, the transfusion should be discontinued.

Transfusion-related acute lung injury

Transfusion-related acute lung injury (TRALI) is a leading cause of transfusion-related mortality in humans and is believed to be widely underrecognized.[24,25] TRALI has the clinical presentation similar to acute respiratory distress syndrome (ARDS) but occurs during or within 6 hours after a transfusion in patients with no preexisting acute lung injury (ALI) before the transfusion. The true incidence in people is unknown and has been reported from all types of blood components. The mortality has been reported to be 5% to 10%. Fresh frozen plasma has been implicated most frequently. In a recent prospective nested case-control study, 74 of 901 (8%) transfused patients developed ALI within 6 hours of transfusion.[24,26] The mechanism of TRALI is not fully understood; however, data from animal models and clinical data suggest immune and nonimmune mechanisms. In the immune mechanism, leukocyte antibodies in the donor react with leukocyte antigens on the recipient neutrophils. The nonimmune mechanism involves insult to the pulmonary vascular endothelium, which results in the activation of cytokines and the release of endothelium adhesion molecules (selectins). This causes neutrophils to adhere to the pulmonary endothelium and a "second hit" causes the release of oxidases and proteases, which damages the pulmonary endothelium and cause vascular leak. TRALI is therefore suspected to be the final common pathway of neutrophil activation and capillary leak.[26]

TRALI has a clinical presentation similar to ARDS occurring in the setting of a transfusion. Signs and symptoms include tachypnea, fever, tachycardia, and hypoxemia, with no evidence of circulatory overload. Central venous pressure is normal. The diagnosis of TRALI is based on a high index of suspicion and requires clinician awareness of the condition. Differentials should therefore include transfusion-associated circulatory overload (TACO), AHTRs, bacterial contamination, and anaphylactoid reactions. TRALI is mainly a diagnosis of exclusion, and the treatment is mainly supportive. Mild cases require supplemental oxygen, whereas severe cases require intravenous fluids and mechanical ventilation. In contrast to ARDS from other causes, TRALI is self-limiting, and human patients usually recover within 96 hours.[24,26]

Acute Nonimmunologic Transfusion Reactions

Transfusion-associated sepsis

In human transfusion medicine, bacterial contamination of blood components accounted for 16% of transfusion-related fatalities reported to the Food and Drug Administration (FDA) between 1986 and 1991 and is considered to be the most common cause of morbidity and mortality related to a transfusion.[27] Bacteria are most often believed to originate in the donor, either from the venipuncture site or from unsuspected bacteremia. Organisms that multiply in refrigerated blood components are psychrophilic gram-negative organisms (eg, Yersinia and Serratia). Gram-positive organisms are more often seen in platelet products stored at room temperature (20°C–24°C). If bacterial contamination is suspected, the transfusion should be stopped immediately and a Gram stain and blood culture should be obtained directly from the unit (not an attached segment of tubing) and the patient. Color change of RBCs, clots, or hemolysis suggests contamination, but the appearance of a contaminated unit can be unremarkable. Care in collection, preparation, and handling of blood components is essential to prevent contamination. If a water bath is used to thaw a component (eg, fresh frozen plasma), use overwrapping to protect the outlet ports from trapping fluid.

Transfusion-associated circulatory overload

Hypervolemia may result from transfusion of whole blood to normovolemic patients or rapid administration of RBCs to normovolemic patients (eg, chronic anemia). In addition, animals with concurrent cardiac or renal compromise may be at risk for TACO. Clinical signs include dyspnea, cyanosis, orthopnea, increased central venous pressure, pulmonary edema, and pulmonary venous distension on thoracic radiographs. Treatment involves discontinuing the transfusion, diuretics, and oxygen.

Nonimmune-mediated hemolysis

RBCs can hemolyze in vitro if the unit is exposed to improper temperatures during shipping or storage or is mishandled at the time of infusion. Malfunctioning blood-warming devices, the use of microwave ovens and hot water baths, or inadvertent freezing may cause temperature-related damage. Mechanical hemolysis can be caused by pressure bags or small bore needles. Osmotic hemolysis may result from the administration of drugs or hypotonic solutions. Prevention involves written procedures for all aspects of collection, processing, storage, and administration of the product. All staff should be trained in the proper use of equipment as well as compatible drugs and intravenous solutions used during administration.

Complications of massive transfusion

Metabolic and hemostatic abnormalities are complications of massive transfusion. Citrate toxicity can occur when large volumes of fresh frozen plasma, whole blood, or platelets are transfused. Plasma citrate levels increase and bind ionized calcium, causing signs of hypocalcemia. Hypothermia can occur from rapid infusion of large volumes of cold blood and may result in ventricular arrhythmias. This is more likely to occur with rapid administration through a central venous catheter and can be avoided by warming blood during massive transfusion. Hyperkalemia and hypokalemia result from RBC storage lesion. Coagulopathies may occur from dilution or loss of platelets and clotting factors.

Air embolism

Air embolism can occur if blood in an open system is infused under pressure or if air enters a central catheter. The minimum volume of air embolism that is potentially fatal for an adult human is 100 mL.[27] Symptoms include cough, dyspnea, and shock. Proper use of infusion pumps and clamping lines while changing tubing prevents this complication.

Delayed Transfusion Reactions

Immune-mediated hemolysis

In a delayed immune-mediated hemolytic transfusion reaction (DHTR), there are no acute clinical signs; however, the patient's posttransfusion packed cell volume (PCV) declines rapidly within 3 to 5 days of the transfusion. Delayed transfusion reactions are caused by the production of RBC antibody shortly after the transfusion of the corresponding antigen. Before the transfusion, these antibodies are present in low titers and not detected by the crossmatch. If a DHTR is suspected, a freshly obtained blood sample from the recipient may be tested for unexpected alloantibodies. Discovery of a new RBC antibody in a recently transfused patient with declining PCV strongly suggests a DHTR, and the diagnosis can be confirmed by demonstrating the corresponding antigen on the transfused RBCs. Future transfusions should lack the antigen responsible for the DHTR even if the antibody becomes undetectable.

SUMMARY

Optimizing patient safety in transfusion medicine is multifaceted. It involves assuring the integrity of the transfusion process from donor collection through posttransfusion evaluation. This facet of human medicine is highly regulated by governmental (eg, FDA) and professional health care organizations (eg, Joint Commission on Accreditation of Healthcare Organizations, American Association of Blood Banks, American Society of Clinical Pathologists). Similar stringency does not currently exist in veterinary medicine; however advances are being made. In 2005, the American College of Veterinary Internal Medicine and the Association of Veterinary Hematology and Transfusion Medicine issued a consensus statement to provide veterinarians guidelines for canine and feline donor screening.[28]

Today, point-of-care tests for blood typing and crossmatching are readily available for dogs and cats. The importance of the pretransfusion testing is to help prevent incompatible RBC transfusions that could lead to immune-mediated transfusion reactions. Blood transfusions are commonly administered to critically ill patients, and although the transfusions themselves can be lifesaving, they are associated with adverse events. Transfusion reactions can be life threatening. The indication for transfusion is a controversial topic in human and veterinary medicine, and the decision of whether or not to transfuse is ultimately made by the attending doctor based on clinical evaluation of patient condition. As veterinary transfusion medicine continues to advance, the transfusion itself needs to be as safe as possible. Mandatory performance of pretransfusion testing improves safety. Furthermore, adverse reactions when they occur should be documented and investigated.

Management and investigation of an acute transfusion reaction

Stop the transfusion; record the volume infused and rate of infusion
Do not discard the blood product, line, or fluids
Verify that the correct blood product is being given to the intended recipient
Examine the unit for hemolysis
Examine the patient for hemolysis
Monitor patient's total physical response, blood pressure, mucous membranes, cardiac resynchronization therapy, and mentation
Retest/recheck blood typing of patient and donor
Crossmatch on a pre- and posttransfusion sample
Chest radiographs and echo, if indicated
Blood cultures.

REFERENCES

1. The immune response, production of antibodies, antigen-antibody reactions. In: Issitt PD, Anstee DJ, editors. Applied blood group serology. 4th edition. Durham (NC): Montgomery Scientific Publications; 1998. p. 15–29.

2. Red cell antigen-antibody reactions and their detection. In: Brecher ME, editor. American association of blood banks technical manual. 15th edition. Bethesda (MD): AABB; 2005. p. 271–6.

3. Hale AS. Canine blood groups and their importance in veterinary medicine. Vet Clin North Am 1995;25:1323–33.

4. Hohenhaus AE. Importance of blood groups and blood group antibodies in companion animal. Transfus Med Rev 2004;18:117–26.

5. Blais MC, Berman L, Oakley DA, et al. Canine Dal blood type: a red cell antigen lacking in some Dalmatians. J Vet Intern Med 2007;21:281–6.

6. Giger U, Gelens CJ, Callan MB, et al. An acute transfusion reaction caused by dog erythrocyte antigen 1.1 incompatibility in a previously sensitized dog. J Am Vet Med Assoc 1995;206:1358–62.

7. Melzer KJ, Wardrop KJ, Hale AS, et al. A hemolytic transfusion reaction due to DEA 4 alloantibodies in a dog. J Vet Intern Med 2003;17:931–3.

8. Auer L, Bell K. The AB blood group system of cats. Anim Blood Groups Biochem Genet 1981;12:287–97.

9. Giger U, Bucheler J, Patterson DF. Frequency and inheritance of A and B blood types in feline breeds in the United States. J Hered 1991;82:15–20.

10. Giger U, Kilrain CG, Filippich LJ, et al. Frequencies of feline blood groups in the United States. J Am Vet Med Assoc 1989;195:1230–2.

11. Knottenbelt CM, Addie DD, Day MJ, et al. Determination of the prevalence of feline blood types in the UK. J Small Anim Pract 1999;40:115–8.

12. Weinstein NM, Blais MC, Harris K, et al. A newly recognized blood group in domestic shorthair cats: the *mik* red cell antigen. J Vet Intern Med 2007;21: 287–92.

13. Bromilow IM, Eggington JA, Owen GA, et al. Red cell anitbody screening and identification: a comparison of two column technology methods. Br J Biomed Sci 1993;50:329–33.

14. Pinkerton PH, Ward J, Couvadia AS. An evaluation of a gel technique for antibody screening compared with a conventional tube method. Transfus Med 1993;3: 201–5.

15. Nathalang O, Chuansumrit A, Prayoonwiwat W, et al. Comparison between the conventional tube technique and the gel technique in direct antiglobulin tests. Vox Sang 1997;72:169–71.

16. Novaretti MCZ, Jens E, Pagliarini T, et al. Comparison of conventional tube test technique and gel microcolumn assay for direct antiglobulin test: a large study. J Clin Lab Anal 2004;18:255–8.

17. Hohenhaus AE, Rentko V. Blood transfusions and blood substitutes, In: DiBartola SP. Editor. Fluid therapy in small animal practice. 3rd edition. St. Louis (MO): Saunders; p. 579–80.

18. Abrams-Ogg A. Practical blood transfusion. In: Day MJ, Mackin A, Littlewood JD, editors. Manual of canine and feline haematology and transfusion medicine. Gloucester (UK): British Small Animal Veterinary Association; 2000. p. 268–75.

19. Lanevschi A, Wardrop KJ. Principles of transfusion medicine in small animals. Can Vet J 2001;42:447–54.

20. Heddle NM. Pathophysiology of febrile nonhemolytic transfusion reactions. Curr Opin Hematol 1999;6:420–6.

21. Geiger TL, Howard SC. Acetaminophen and diphenhydramine premedication for allergic and febrile non-hemolytic transfusion reactions: good prophylaxis or bad practice. Transfus Med Rev 2007;21(1):1–12.

22. Bracker KE, Drellich S. Transfusion reactions. Compendium 2005;501–12.

23. Noninfectious complications of blood transfusion. In: Brecher ME, editor. American association of blood banks technical manual. 15th edition. Bethesda (MD): AABB; 2005. p. 644–7.

24. Gajic O, Rana R, Winters JL, et al. Transfusion-related acute lung injury in the critically ill. Am J Respir Crit Care Med 2007;176:886–91.

25. O'Quinn RJ, Lakshminarayan S. Venous air embolism. Arch Intern Med 1892;142: 2173–6.

26. Triulzi DJ. Transfusion-related acute lung injury: an update. Hematology Am Soc Hematol Educ Program 2006;497–501.

27. Brecher ME, editor. American association of blood banks technical manual. 15th edition. Bethesda (MD): AABB; 2005. p. 651, 652, 691, 692.

28. Wardrop KJ, Reine N, Birkenheuer A, et al. Canine and feline blood donor screening for infectious disease. J Vet Intern Med 2005;19:135–42.

Transplantation in Small Animals

Barrak M. Pressler, DVM, PhD

KEYWORDS

- Dog • Cat • Transplantation • Immunology
- Rejection • Kidney

Transplantation of tissues and parenchymal organs has become an accepted treatment modality in people over the last half century. However, despite the much more limited use of transplantation in veterinary medicine, the first reported organ transplants were performed in dogs in the early twentieth century.[1,2] These early transplants were followed by studies in experimental animals that demonstrated the comparative success of organ transplants from animals of the same versus different species, and refined many of the surgical techniques that are in place today.[3] In fact, the initial work that developed many of the vascular suture techniques still in use was performed in dogs, and in conjunction with his studies on preservation of explanted organs, led to Alexis Carrel being awarded the Nobel Prize in Medicine in 1912.[1,3] The introduction of new immunosuppressive drugs, particularly cyclosporine, in the 1980s vastly improved short- and long-term outcomes of transplanted tissues, and thus reduced morbidity and mortality of transplant recipients. The United States Department of Health and Human Services now reports that human kidney, heart, cornea, and bone marrow transplants all have 5-year graft survival rates greater than or equal to 70%, and transplantation of these four organs is collectively performed in more than 70,000 patients per year in the United States alone.[4]

TRANSPLANTATION IMMUNOLOGY
Transplant Terminology: Auto-, Iso-, Allo-, and Xenografts

Transplanted tissue may be harvested from a variety of sources. Tissues or organs harvested from one location and reimplanted in the same patient in a new location are termed autografts. Autografts most commonly used in human and veterinary patients are skin transplants for repair of large wounds (eg, following excision of large nonviable burns or cutaneous masses) and cortical bone (in order to provide scaffolding and osteoblasts where needed). Isografts, also called syngeneic grafts, are tissue transplants between genetically identical individuals, such as between monozygotic twins or unrelated mice from the same inbred strain. Allografts are tissue or

Department of Veterinary Clinical Sciences, School of Veterinary Medicine, Purdue University, Lynn Hall, 625 Harrison Street, West Lafayette, IN 47907, USA
E-mail address: barrak@purdue.edu

Vet Clin Small Anim 40 (2010) 495–505
doi:10.1016/j.cvsm.2010.01.005   **vetsmall.theclinics.com**

organ transplants between unrelated or related but genetically different individuals from the same species. The vast majority of transplants in human and veterinary medicine (including transplants from one family member to another, from unrelated individuals to each other, and from cadavers or living donors) are allografts. Xenografts are tissue or organ transplants derived from a different species than the recipient.

Major Histocompatibility Complex Proteins

A complete discussion of the mechanisms whereby the immune system recognizes cells and proteins as belonging to the host (ie, recognition of self) and how autoimmune reactions are inhibited or curtailed, whereas foreign proteins and microbes elicit an immune response, is beyond the scope of this article. However, to understand the concepts of tissue-matching and rejection, a brief overview of immunologic surveillance follows. The reader should refer to a general immunology textbook for a more thorough discussion of identification of self, maintenance of tolerance, and elimination of auto-reactive lymphocytes from the systemic repertoire.

Those microbes that successfully penetrate the host's natural barriers (ie, skin and mucosa) usually first elicit a response via activation of the innate immune system. Unlike the adaptive immune response (see the discussion later in this article), the innate immune system is an umbrella term for those cells, soluble proteins, and cell-surface receptors that recognize large classes of microbes, are capable of rapid response, do not have the ability to increase their specificity over time, are not interdependent, and lack memory. Examples of cellular components of the innate immune system include (but are by no means limited to) neutrophils and natural killer cells, whereas example circulating proteins and cell-surface receptors include the complement cascade, antiviral interferons, and Toll-like receptors. Although critical for initiating immune responses to foreign antigens, the innate immune system plays little role in tolerance or rejection of transplanted tissues.

The adaptive immune response refers to the interdependent presentation of self- and foreign-derived peptides by major histocompatibility complex (MHC) proteins, surveillance of these cell-surface protein-peptide complexes by T-lymphocytes, and activation of effector T- and B- lymphocytes capable of clonal expansion into cytotoxic, helper, and antibody-producing cells. Maturing T-cells traverse the thymus, during which any cells which express T-cell receptors that fail to bind or conversely strongly bind host MHC molecules in the absence of an MHC-displayed peptide, or which bind host MHC molecules which display host protein-derived peptides (ie, self-reactive lymphocytes), are eliminated. The remaining T-lymphocyte repertoire therefore is composed only of those cells which weakly bind host MHC molecules, and do not react with host peptides.

MHC-I proteins are expressed by all nucleated cells and display peptides derived from any protein produced by a particular cell's own translational machinery. Circulating $CD8^+$ T cells survey peptides being displayed by these MHC-I proteins; host peptides for the most part should not elicit an immune response, whereas virus-derived peptides (which in many cases are displayed by MHC-I molecules, as they are produced after viral hijacking of the host cell machinery) elicit a cytotoxic response against the infected cells. MHC-II proteins, in contrast, are predominantly displayed by dendritic cells, macrophages, and B-cells, collectively known as antigen-presenting cells (APCs). Following receptor-mediated phagocytosis of antigens, APCs degrade the internalized proteins and display the resultant peptides on MHC-II molecules to lymphocytes in lymph nodes and the spleen. In addition, APCs become sensitized by an inflammatory cytokine milieu such that they alter surface expression of co-stimulatory proteins, which are required to induce an immune response. When a CD4$^+$ T-cell displaying a T-cell receptor that recognizes the host MHC-II molecule bound to a foreign peptide comes in contact with the APC, and the APC has been sensitized and can provide a 'second signal', via co-stimulatory proteins, then clonal expansion of the CD4$^+$ T-cell occurs, and either a T_H1- or T_H2-dominant response is induced. Phagocytosis of antigen by APCs without concurrent activation by inflammatory cytokines may still result in T-cell/MHC/peptide binding, but absence of the co-stimulatory molecule second signal leads to T-cell anergy. Anergy is not merely a lack of response but a state of non-responsiveness (ie, the T cell becomes unable to respond to antigen recognition).

Despite the unimaginably large number of possible peptides derivable from foreign and host proteins, mammalian genomes characterized thus far contain only a limited number of MHC proteins that are co-dominantly expressed. For example, in people there are three MHC-I gene loci on chromosome 6, and therefore a maximum of six different MHC-I proteins expressed on nucleated cells (three from each of the chromosome 6 pair); likewise, human beings express a maximum of six different MHC-II proteins. Because hundreds of alleles have been characterized at these loci, as an example, five unrelated individuals could easily have amongst them thirty different MHC-I proteins.

Graft Rejection

Rejection of transplanted organs occurs when, despite prior tissue cross-matching and administration of immunosuppressive drugs, the recipient's immune system recognizes the donor tissue as foreign. Anti-graft immune responses are invariably caused by an acquired immune response. Although immune response terminology (hyperacute, acute, or chronic) somewhat approximates the length of time posttransplantation that rejection occurs, it more accurately refers to the infiltrating cell type and pathologic findings noted on examination of tissue.

Rejection may be associated with anti-graft antibodies or T cells. Although MHC molecules are normally responsible for maintenance of tolerance, it is the allogeneic MHC molecules expressed on grafted tissues and transported donor leukocytes that are usually recognized as foreign by the recipient's immune system and induce graft rejection. In fact, this is how MHC molecules were first named; the ability of MHC molecules to induce graft rejection (ie, to determine histocompatibility) was recognized before their role in recognition of self and immunologic surveillance was elucidated. As a result, determining which MHC alleles are present within a given patient and attempting to transplant organs from individuals that are ideally identical at all loci is always attempted in people. This process is referred to as tissue typing, and is critical because closer MHC matching of donor and recipient significantly decreases the likelihood of rejection; however, inexact donor-recipient MHC matches must still be performed because the number of available organs is far lower than the number of patients awaiting transplants.

Hyperacute rejection

Hyperacute rejection occurs when the recipient has preexisting circulating antibodies against antigens displayed by transplant cells, particularly by graft endothelial cells. This may occur because of previous transplantations (for example, individuals with a second renal transplant following rejection of the first transplant); blood transfusions; or when xenografts are used. Blood type cross-matching before human, canine, or feline allograft transplantation (accompanied by MHC matching before human or canine allograft transplantation) vastly decreases the incidence of hyperacute rejection. However, because antibodies that react with xenograft endothelial cell antigens appear to be inherently present in most mammalian species, and xenograft cells lack species-specific regulatory proteins that prevent fixation of complement, the chronic shortage in transplantable organs has thus far not been overcome by relying on more readily available xenograft tissues. Antibody binding of foreign antigens during hyperacute graft rejection results in organ-wide complement activation, endothelial cell damage, and exposure of sub-endothelial basement membrane components leading to extravasation of activated inflammatory cells and thrombosis of vessels secondary to initiation of the clotting cascade. Surgeons may note engorgement and discoloration of transplanted organs in cases of hyperacute rejection within minutes after anastomosis of donor and recipient blood vessels.

Acute rejection

As the name implies, acute rejection may occur within days of transplantation, but when immunosuppressive drugs are administered, this form of graft failure may still be noted months following implantation of foreign tissue. Recognition of graft-derived peptides in a naïve (ie, no preexisting activated anti-graft T cells or circulating antibodies) recipient may occur by two mechanisms. So-called direct allorecognition occurs when donor APCs that were present within the allograft tissue enter the recipient's circulation, travel to lymph nodes, and present peptides to the recipient's lymphocytes. Direct allorecognition occurs because the donor APCs are not only presenting peptides in the context of foreign MHC molecules but because they also possess co-stimulatory activity that activates the host immune response. Indirect allorecognition occurs when graft-derived proteins are phagocytized and presented by the recipient's own APCs. Although graft MHC-derived peptides may initiate indirect allorecognition, minor H antigens are more commonly implicated. H antigens are peptides derived from the myriad of other cellular proteins that are not donor-recipient tissue matched before transplantation, with some examples being Y-chromosome translated proteins when transplanted into female patients, and the Rh protein in human blood transfusions. Direct allorecognition most commonly results in a CD8+ T-cell-mediated rejection response, particularly when the MHC-I molecules are recognized as foreign with or without graft-derived peptides being displayed, and indirect allorecognition usually results in a CD4+ T-cell-mediated rejection response (often with accompanying antibody production) caused by recognition of graft-derived peptides in the context of recipient MHC-II molecules.

Graft histologic change findings that are consistent with acute rejection depend on the antigen that has initiated the immune response. For example, in human renal allografts, 45% to 70% of acute T-cell–mediated rejections result in a primarily tubulointerstitial pattern of inflammation, 30% to 55% in a vascular pattern, and 2% to 4% in a glomerular pattern.[5] Histopathologic examination typically reveals activated T-cell and monocyte infiltration in cases of cellular rejection, whereas antibody-mediated rejection more commonly leads to neutrophil infiltration and fibrinoid necrosis of arteries.[5] In people with acute rejection of renal allografts, immunofluorescent detection of deposition of the activated component of C4 (known as C4d) is a sensitive and specific method for differentiating between cellular and acute rejection.[6,7] Differentiation of antibody- versus T-cell–mediated acute rejection may be important because in theory, optimal therapy may differ. For example, in human renal transplant recipients, plasmapheresis and anti–B-cell therapies (such as mycophenolate mofetil) may be of more use in antibody-mediated rejection episodes, whereas high-dose steroids and anti–T-cell monoclonal antibody therapy are standardly used for T-cell–mediated acute rejection.[5]

The likelihood that patients will suffer an acute rejection episode decreases over time. Studies of protocol biopsies (see later discussion) from human renal transplant recipients have suggested that an initial acceptance reaction, during which graft infiltrates increase but inflammatory cell activation decreases (ie, reduction in CD3[+] T-cells, decreased CD25[+] expression, and increased T-cell apoptosis) may precede an accommodation state during which immunosuppressive drugs are sufficient to prevent progression of histologic changes consistent with rejection.[5] Biomolecular changes associated with accommodation may include downregulation or internalization of rejection-associated donor cell antigens, and repopulation of the donated organ's endothelium with recipient cells.[5] True tolerance, whereby graft organs remain viable after withdrawal of all immunosuppressive therapy, is rare.

Chronic rejection

Chronic rejection develops over months or years following transplantation; for example, chronic rejection develops in 2% to 5% of human renal transplants each year, with the half-life of renal transplants limited to approximately 8 years.[4] The pathogenesis of chronic rejection is likely similar to that of acute rejection, with anti-allogeneic MHC immune responses oftentimes resulting in anti-graft T-cells or antibodies. Those histologic changes previously described in acutely rejected tissues can also be found in cases of chronic rejection, but fibrosis, arteriosclerosis, basement membrane duplication, and circulating anti-MHC antibodies predominate over hemorrhage, necrosis, and neutrophil infiltration. Why it is that despite presumptively identical immune initiators some patients develop acute rejection whereas others develop chronic rejection is unclear; contributing factors may include the closeness of MHC matching; degree of polymorphism in recipient versus graft MHC and H antigen proteins; ischemia-reperfusion injury; recurrence of the initial disease in the transplanted organ, and in the case of renal transplants, calcineurin inhibitor toxicity. Chronic rejection carries a worse prognosis for most organs than acute rejection, and transplantation with a new organ is often eventually required.

Graft-versus-host Disease

Graft-versus-host disease occurs in bone marrow transplant recipients. Following ablation of the recipient's bone marrow (usually by high-dose cytotoxic drugs or whole-body irradiation), progenitor cells are repopulated using cells from an MHC-matched donor. Although the goal of bone marrow transplantation is usually to provide the recipient with non-neoplastic stem cells (in the case of patients with leukemia) or with immunocompetent cells (in those patients with congenital immunodeficiencies), mature T-cells are oftentimes inadvertently transferred from the donor as well. These T-cells enter the recipient's circulation, come in contact with host APCs that present peptides in the context of MHC molecules, and are activated by the same mechanisms described earlier in direct allorecognition. Clonal expansion of these activated lymphocytes leads to systemic inflammation, with common clinical signs including erythema/rashes, pneumonitis, and diarrhea.

CURRENT STATUS OF TRANSPLANTATION IN VETERINARY MEDICINE

Blood is by far the most commonly transplanted tissue in veterinary medicine; for a thorough discussion of transfusion medicine, please refer to the article elsewhere in this issue. Other than blood, routine transplantation of allograft or xenograft tissues is still quite limited in small animal veterinary medicine. The only parenchymal organ that can be said to be routinely transplanted in client-owned small animals is allograft kidneys in cats. Of the possible non-parenchymal organ transplantations, allo- and xenograft corneal transplantations are well described, and bone marrow transplantation has been used as an adjunct to kidney transplantation or treatment of hematopoietic tumors in dogs.

Renal Transplantation

Kidney allograft transplantation is a successful treatment modality for cats with end-stage kidney disease. The first successful feline kidney transplantation was performed in 1987 at the University of California, Davis, School of Veterinary Medicine.[8,9] Several hundred successful kidney allograft transplants have since been performed in cats, but unfortunately this procedure is currently offered at less than 10 sites in the United States.[10] In a study of 66 cats receiving kidney transplants, 71% of cats survived until discharge.[11] One-year survival rate in this early case series was 51%, but advances in surgical technique have since resulted in greater survival times.[12–14] The most commonly identified pathologic conditions for which kidney transplantation is performed include chronic interstitial nephritis (48%), polycystic kidneys (10%), ethylene glycol toxicosis (9%), and renal fibrosis (6%).[11] Because of the morbidity, mortality, and expense associated with transplantation, candidate patients are typically limited to those whose renal function continues to decompensate despite aggressive supportive and symptomatic medical management.

Unfortunately, although kidney allograft transplantation has also been successfully performed in dogs, transplantation in this species presents a greater challenge because of the level of immunosuppression required to prevent allograft rejection.[15,16] Rejection episodes in dogs are frequent and severe, and canine recipients require multiple-agent immunosuppressive protocols and intensive management.[16,17] Several studies have explored triple-drug (cyclosporine, azathioprine, and prednisolone) protocols and histocompatibility matching with limited success; therefore, to date, high complication and mortality rates in dogs preclude widespread use of kidney transplantation for treatment of renal failure in this species.[16,17]

Thorough discussion of the medical management, screening, and anesthetic and surgical aspects of renal transplantation in cats is beyond the scope of this article and has been recently reviewed elsewhere.[10,18] However, in brief, once thorough screening eliminates those patients with comorbid conditions that significantly increase peri- and postoperative morbidity and mortality, preoperative management generally includes parenteral fluid diuresis, treatment with recombinant human erythropoietin or blood transfusions to achieve a hematocrit greater than 30%, and initiation of immunosuppressive therapy.[10,19] Despite the previously described concerns regarding MHC matching in human transplantation medicine, tissue typing is not routinely performed in cats; current immunosuppressive protocols have minimized rejection episodes such that kidneys from unrelated, non–MHC-matched donors can be tolerated for years.[10,18]

At the time of surgery the donor kidney is removed through a ventral midline celiotomy, with the left kidney preferred because of the increased length of the vascular pedicle. Although several techniques for vascular anastomosis and ureteral implantation have been described, anastomosis of the donor kidney vessels to the postrenal aorta and vena cava,[20] extra-vesicular ureteroneocystostomy,[21] and mucosal apposition of the ureter to the bladder are recommended.[10,18] The recipient's kidneys are left in place and only removed at a later date if necessary.

Renal function and hemodynamic parameters typically return to normal within 3 to 5 days after transplantation.[11] Reported immediate postoperative complications include acute graft rejection, hypertension,[22] and neurologic signs,[23,24] although current immunosuppressive protocols have vastly decreased the incidence of acute rejection episodes. Nineteen presumptive episodes of allograft rejection were noted in 12 out of

66 (18%) cats, most commonly in the first 2 months after surgery.[11] If the transplant recipient remains anorectic or serum creatinine concentration continues to rise with production of minimally concentrated urine following surgery, then graft rejection should be suspected. Antirejection therapy in cats consists of methylprednisolone sodium succinate, with some transplant centers also administering intravenous cyclosporine to maintain therapeutic serum concentrations.[10,18] Severe postoperative hypertension requiring intervention (systolic blood pressure >170 mm Hg) has been reported in 62% of recipient cats.[22] Central nervous system disorders have been reported in 21% of cats receiving transplants, with seizures occurring in 88% of these cases, but successful management of hypertension reduces the prevalence of these neurologic complications.[22,24]

Organ transplant recipients must be maintained on lifelong immunosuppressive therapy,[10,25] with some transplant institutions beginning cyclosporine administration 2 weeks before surgery to ensure adequate serum trough levels at the time of surgery, thus preventing possible early initiation of an anti-graft immune response.[10,18] In the absence of immunosuppression, transplanted kidney allografts from unrelated, histo-incompatible cat donors are rejected within 5 to 8 days.[26]

In people, suspected renal transplant rejection episodes are routinely confirmed via biopsy of the transplanted organ. Renal biopsy results alter the clinical diagnosis in approximately one third of patients with suspected rejection, and result in a change in recommended therapy in almost 60% of transplant recipients.[5] Histopathologic findings consistent with antibody-mediated rejection include C4d deposition, acute tubular necrosis-like inflammation, and thromboses.[5] T-cell–mediated rejection episodes, which may occur in concert with antibody-mediated rejection, usually are associated with mononuclear cell infiltration, tubulitis, intimal arteritis, and fibrosis.[5] Despite the value of indication biopsies in human patients, biopsies are not commonly performed in feline renal transplant recipients with increased serum creatinine concentrations because urine specific gravity, aerobic urine culture, abdominal ultrasound, and whole blood cyclosporine concentrations frequently are sufficient for excluding or making a presumptive diagnosis of acute rejection in cats. Rejection is frequently associated with subtherapeutic whole blood cyclosporine concentrations,[14] and because calcineurin inhibitor toxicity (a common cause of renal failure in human renal transplant recipients) is of unknown significance in cats, there is less call for renal biopsy to differentiate this condition from suspected rejection. A single retrospective review of renal biopsies and allograft kidneys obtained after euthanasia of client-owned feline transplant recipients revealed that the lesions most commonly noted differ from those in people.[27] Using the Banff 1997 classification[5] (the standard algorithm by which human nephropathologists grade transplant rejection-associated lesions), the most common abnormalities indicating active or acute lesions were mild to moderate tubulitis (53% of specimens); polymorphonuclear glomerular infiltrate (ie, necrotizing glomerulonephritis; 25%); and lymphocytic phlebitis of large veins (48%). In people, phlebitis is sufficiently rare that it is not included in the 1997 classification, whereas monocytic arteritis, which is routinely noted, was not present in any of the 77 specimens evaluated.[27]

In addition to indication biopsies, protocol biopsies are also performed by most human renal transplant centers at predetermined intervals to identify inflammatory histologic changes consistent with rejection, but before overt graft dysfunction occurs. Approximately 15% of human transplant recipients may have subclinical acute rejection within 6 months of surgery, and slightly more than 20% have inflammatory changes that are considered suspicious for rejection.[5] In the study mentioned earlier examining transplants from feline patients, the most common lesions noted were mild to moderate fibrosis (60% of specimens); mild to moderate tubular atrophy (45%); and mild to moderate increases in mesangial matrix (45%). Sixty-nine percent of samples had histologic lesions consistent with chronic allograft nephropathy.[27] In dogs with mismatched MHC renal allografts and concurrent bone marrow transplantation, a majority of animals demonstrated mild lymphoplasmacytic peritubular inflammation, whereas following tapering of immunosuppressive drugs, most had moderate to severe perivascular and peritubular lymphoplasmacytic inflammation with variable tubulitis and tubular atrophy that accompanied worsening azotemia.[28]

Long-term adverse effects in feline renal transplant recipients include an increased incidence of infections (particularly urinary tract infections)[14,29,30]; neoplasia (with lymphoproliferative neoplasms being diagnosed most frequently)[31,32]; and diabetes mellitus.[33] Although killed/inactivated or recombinant/subunit vaccines have been anecdotally advocated in transplant recipients over attenuated/modified-live products, there have been no studies investigating whether vaccine type influences development of infectious disease.

Corneal Transplantation (Keratoplasty)

The anterior chamber and cornea are immunologically privileged sites. Although antigens are taken up by resident APCs that enter the systemic circulation and present peptides to T-lymphocytes, the resultant immune reaction is one of tolerance and downregulation, rather than induction of inflammation.[34] This process, known as anterior chamber-associated immune deviation, has thus far allowed allograft corneal transplantation in dogs and cats without concurrent immunosuppressive therapy.[34] Transplantation of fresh corneas and corneas that have undergone short-term storage[35,36] has been performed for a variety of conditions, including melting ulcers and following partial keratectomy for treatment of sequestra or neoplasms.[37,38] Anterior chamber-associated immune deviation also permits tolerance of xenograft transplantations, not only of corneal tissue from other species (usually dog corneas to cat recipients)[38,39] but also of alternative tissues, such as equine or porcine amniotic membrane[40,41] or porcine small intestinal submucosa,[42–44] which are more widely available and of the approximate thickness and transparency of the normal cornea. However, although immunosuppressive medications are not used following keratoplasty in small animals, up to 30% of corneal grafts in people undergo at least one rejection episode.[45] Larger case series with more systematic evaluation, including histologic evaluation, are needed before it can be definitively stated that tolerance following keratoplasty is absolute in dogs and cats.

Bone Marrow Transplantation

Reports of bone marrow transplantation in client-owned small animals are limited to autologous transplants as part of a myeloablative protocol for treatment of lymphoma in dogs,[46–49] and as allograft transplants in dogs with lymphoma[50] or in conjunction with renal transplantation in an attempt to improve long-term tolerance. Lymphoma or leukemia treatment protocols that incorporate bone marrow transplantation into multidrug chemotherapy protocols have thus far not improved survival rates beyond those using chemotherapy alone.[47–49] Rationale for combining bone marrow with renal transplantation in dogs is because, as previously mentioned, the level of immunosuppression required to prevent kidney allograft rejection in this species frequently results in severe, intolerable side effects. Concurrent bone marrow transplantation induces immunologic chimerism in dogs (ie, transplanted dogs are provided with donor lymphocyte stem cells that traverse the thymus, mature, and are not activated via direct allorecognition).[51,52] However, because indirect allorecognition caused by recipient T-lymphocyte recognition of H antigen peptides still occurs, lifelong immuno-suppressive therapy is still required.[52]

SUMMARY

Advances in surgical techniques and immunosuppressive therapy have allowed trans-plantations to become a widely used therapy in people with failure of a variety of organs. Cell surface proteins, which mediate tolerance and eventual rejection of organs, particularly in the kidney, have been well characterized in people. Neverthe-less, despite the relative conservation of the acquired immune response in mammals, for unknown reasons dogs and cats either tolerate more readily or reject more vigor-ously transplanted organs. In addition, although several rejection-associated histo-logic changes are found in human and animal grafts, differences imply that the immune response to graft proteins nevertheless is not identical amongst species. As of now, very few tissues or organs are routinely transplanted in client-owned dogs and cats, and larger studies are still needed to characterize chronic changes that may develop. With the continual development of new immunosuppressive drugs and refinement of existing protocols, transplantation options will hopefully increase, particularly in dogs, and via the use of xenograft tissues.

REFERENCES

1. Carrel A. Transplantation in mass of the kidneys. J Exp Med 1908;10:98–140.
2. Ullmann E. Experimentelle Nierentransplantation [Experimental kidney trans-plantation]. Wien Klin Wochenschr 1902;15:281 [in German].
3. Carrel A. La technique operatoire des anastamoses vasculaires et la transplanta-tion des visceres [A surgical technique for vascular anastamosis and organ transplantation]. Lyon Med 1902;98:859 [in French].
4. U.S. Organ Procurement and Transplantation Network and Scientific Registry of Transplant Recipients Annual Report. In: Shevrin CA, editor. OPTN/SRTR annual report. Washington, DC: U.S. Department of Health and Human Services; 2008.
5. Colvin RB, Nickeleit V. Renal transplant pathology. In: Jennette JC, Olson JL, Schwartz MM, Silva FG, editors. Heptinstall's pathology of the kidney. Hagers-town (MD): Lippincott Williams & Wilkins; 2006. p. 1347–490.
6. Feucht HE, Mihatsch MJ. Diagnostic value of C4d in renal biopsies. Curr Opin Nephrol Hypertens 2005;14:592–8.
7. Nickeleit V, Zeiler M, Gudat F, et al. Detection of the complement degradation product C4d in renal allografts: diagnostic and therapeutic implications. J Am Soc Nephrol 2002;13:242–51.
8. Gregory CR, Gourley IM, Kochin EJ, et al. Renal transplantation for treatment of end-stage renal failure in cats. J Am Vet Med Assoc 1992;201:285–91.
9. Gregory CR, Gourley IM, Taylor NJ, et al. Preliminary results of clinical renal allo-graft transplantation in the dog and cat. J Vet Intern Med 1987;1:53–60.
10. Bleedorn JA, Pressler BM. Screening and medical management of feline kidney transplant candidates. Vet Med 2008;103:92–103.
11. Mathews KG, Gregory CR. Renal transplants in cats: 66 cases (1987–1996). J Am Vet Med Assoc 1997;211:1432–6.
12. Aronson LR, Kyles AE, Preston A, et al. Renal transplantation in cats with calcium oxalate urolithiasis: 19 cases (1997–2004). J Am Vet Med Assoc 2006;228:743–9.
13. Mehl ML, Kyles AE, Pollard R, et al. Comparison of 3 techniques for ureteroneo-cystostomy in cats. Vet Surg 2005;34:114–9.

14. Schmiedt CW, Holzman G, Schwarz T, et al. Survival, complications, and analysis of risk factors after renal transplantation in cats. Vet Surg 2008;37:683–95.

15. Gregory CR, Gourley IM, Haskins SC, et al. Effects of mizoribine on canine renal allograft recipients. Am J Vet Res 1988;49:305–11.

16. Gregory CR, Kyles AE, Bernsteen L, et al. Results of clinical renal transplantation in 15 dogs using triple drug immunosuppressive therapy. Vet Surg 2006;35: 105–12.

17. Mathews KA, Holmberg DL, Miller CW. Kidney transplantation in dogs with naturally occurring end-stage renal disease. J Am Anim Hosp Assoc 2000;36: 294–301.

18. Adin CA. Renal transplantation. In: Bonagura JD, Twedt DC, editors. Kirk's current veterinary therapy XIV. St. Louis (MO): Saunders Elsevier; 2008. p. 901–6.

19. Katayama M, McAnulty JF. Renal transplantation in cats: patient selection and preoperative management. Compendium on Continuing Education for the Small Animal Practitioner 2002;24:868–73.

20. Bernsteen L, Gregory CR, Pollard RE, et al. Comparison of two surgical techniques for renal transplantation in cats. Vet Surg 1999;28:417–20.

21. Kochin EJ, Gregory CR, Wisner E, et al. Evaluation of a method of ureteroneocystostomy in cats. J Am Vet Med Assoc 1993;202:257–60.

22. Kyles AE, Gregory CR, Wooldridge JD, et al. Management of hypertension controls postoperative neurologic disorders after renal transplantation in cats. Vet Surg 1999;28:436–41.

23. Adin CA, Gregory CR, Kyles AE, et al. Diagnostic predictors of complications and survival after renal transplantation in cats. Vet Surg 2001;30:515–21.

24. Gregory CR, Mathews KG, Aronson LR, et al. Central nervous system disorders after renal transplantation in cats. Vet Surg 1997;26:386–92.

25. Bernsteen L, Gregory CR, Kyles AE, et al. Renal transplantation in cats. Clin Tech Small Anim Pract 2000;15:40–5.

26. Kyles AE, Gregory CR, Griffey SM, et al. Evaluation of the clinical and histologic features of renal allograft rejection in cats. Vet Surg 2002;31:49–56.

27. De Cock HE, Kyles AE, Griffey SM, et al. Histopathologic findings and classification of feline renal transplants. Vet Pathol 2004;41:244–56.

28. Broaddus KD, Tillson DM, Lenz SD, et al. Renal allograft histopathology in dog leukocyte antigen mismatched dogs after renal transplantation. Vet Surg 2006; 35:125–35.

29. Nordquist BC, Aronson LR. Pyogranulomatous cystitis associated with Toxoplasma gondii infection in a cat after renal transplantation. J Am Vet Med Assoc 2008;232:1010–2.

30. Kadar E, Sykes JE, Kass PH, et al. Evaluation of the prevalence of infections in cats after renal transplantation: 169 cases (1987–2003). J Am Vet Med Assoc 2005;227:948–53.

31. Schmiedt CW, Grimes JA, Holzman G, et al. Incidence and risk factors for development of malignant neoplasia after feline renal transplantation and cyclosporine-based immunosuppression. Vet Comp Oncol 2009;7:45–53.

32. Wooldridge JD, Gregory CR, Mathews KG, et al. The prevalence of malignant neoplasia in feline renal-transplant recipients. Vet Surg 2002;31:94–7.

33. Case JB, Kyles AE, Nelson RW, et al. Incidence of and risk factors for diabetes mellitus in cats that have undergone renal transplantation: 187 cases (1986–2005). J Am Vet Med Assoc 2007;230:880–4.

34. Biros D. Anterior chamber-associated immune deviation. Vet Clin North Am Small Anim Pract 2008;38:309–21, vi–vii.

35. Arndt C, Reese S, Kostlin R. Preservation of canine and feline corneoscleral tissue in optisol GS. Vet Ophthalmol 2001;4:175–82.
36. Dice PF 2nd, Severin GA, Lumb WV. Experimental autogenous and homologous corneal transplantation in the dog. J Am Anim Hosp Assoc 1973;9:245–51.
37. Norman JC, Urbanz JL, Calvarese ST. Penetrating keratoscleroplasty and bimodal grafting for treatment of limbal melanocytoma in a dog. Vet Ophthalmol 2008;11:340–5.
38. Pena Gimenez MT, Farina IM. Lamellar keratoplasty for the treatment of feline corneal sequestrum. Vet Ophthalmol 1998;1:163–5.
39. Townsend WM, Rankin AJ, Stiles J, et al. Heterologous penetrating keratoplasty for treatment of a corneal sequestrum in a cat. Vet Ophthalmol 2008;11:273–8.
40. Barros PS, Safatle AM, Godoy CA, et al. Amniotic membrane transplantation for the reconstruction of the ocular surface in three cases. Vet Ophthalmol 2005;8: 189–92.
41. Tsuzuki K, Yamashita K, Izumisawa Y, et al. Microstructure and glycosaminoglycan ratio of canine cornea after reconstructive transplantation with glycerin-preserved porcine amniotic membranes. Vet Ophthalmol 2008;11:222–7.
42. Bussieres M, Krohne SG, Stiles J, et al. The use of porcine small intestinal submucosa for the repair of full-thickness corneal defects in dogs, cats and horses. Vet Ophthalmol 2004;7:352–9.
43. Lewin GA. Repair of a full thickness corneoscleral defect in a German shepherd dog using porcine small intestinal submucosa. J Small Anim Pract 1999;40: 340–2.
44. Vanore M, Chahory S, Payen G, et al. Surgical repair of deep melting ulcers with porcine small intestinal submucosa (SIS) graft in dogs and cats. Vet Ophthalmol 2007;10:93–9.
45. Panda A, Vanathi M, Kumar A, et al. Corneal graft rejection. Surv Ophthalmol 2007;52:375–96.
46. Appelbaum FR, Deeg HJ, Storb R, et al. Cure of malignant lymphoma in dogs with peripheral blood stem cell transplantation. Transplantation 1986;42:19–22.
47. Bowles CA, Bull M, McCormick K, et al. Autologous bone marrow transplantation following chemotherapy and irradiation in dogs with spontaneous lymphomas. J Natl Cancer Inst 1980;65:615–20.
48. Deeg HJ, Appelbaum FR, Weiden PL, et al. Autologous marrow transplantation as consolidation therapy for canine lymphoma: efficacy and toxicity of various regimens of total body irradiation. Am J Vet Res 1985;46:2016–8.
49. Frimberger AE, Moore AS, Rassnick KM, et al. A combination chemotherapy protocol with dose intensification and autologous bone marrow transplant (VEL-CAP-HDC) for canine lymphoma. J Vet Intern Med 2006;20:355–64.
50. Lupu M, Sullivan EW, Westfall TE, et al. Use of multigeneration-family molecular dog leukocyte antigen typing to select a hematopoietic cell transplant donor for a dog with T-cell lymphoma. J Am Vet Med Assoc 2006;228:728–32.
51. Graves SS, Hogan WJ, Kuhr C, et al. Adoptive immunotherapy against allogeneic kidney grafts in dogs with stable hematopoietic trichimerism. Biol Blood Marrow Transplant 2008;14:1201–8.
52. Tillson M, Niemeyer GP, Welch JA, et al. Hematopoietic chimerism induces renal and skin allograft tolerance in DLA-identical dogs. Exp Hematol 2006;34: 1759–70.

Cancer Immunotherapy

Philip J. Bergman, DVM, MS, PhD[a,b],*

KEYWORDS

- Cancer • Vaccine • Immunotherapy • Tumor

The term immunity is derived from the Latin word immunitas, which refers to the legal protection afforded to Roman senators holding office. Although the immune system provides protection against infectious disease (and much of this issue of *Veterinary Clinics of North America* is devoted to this), the ability of the immune system to recognize and eliminate cancer is the fundamental rationale for immunotherapy for cancer. Multiple lines of evidence support a role for the immune system in managing cancer, including (1) spontaneous remissions in cancer patients without treatment; (2) the presence of tumor-specific cytotoxic T cells within tumors or draining lymph nodes; (3) the presence of monocytic, lymphocytic, and plasmacytic cellular infiltrates in tumors; (4) the increased incidence of some types of cancer in immunosuppressed patients; and (5) documentation of cancer remissions with the use of immunomodulators.[1,2] With the tools of molecular biology and a greater understanding of mechanisms to harness the immune system, effective tumor immunotherapy is becoming a reality. This new class of therapeutics offers a more targeted, and therefore precise, approach to the treatment of cancer. It is likely that immunotherapy will have a place alongside the classic cancer treatment triad components of surgery, radiation therapy, and chemotherapy within the next 5 to 10 years.

TUMOR IMMUNOLOGY
Cellular Components

The immune system is generally divided into 2 primary components: the innate immune response, and the highly specific but more slowly developing adaptive or acquired immune response. Innate immunity is rapidly acting but typically not specific and includes physicochemical barriers (eg, skin and mucosa), blood proteins such as complement, phagocytic cells (macrophages, neutrophils, dendritic cells [DCs], and natural killer [NK] cells), and cytokines that coordinate and regulate the cells involved in innate immunity. Adaptive immunity is considered to be the acquired arm of immunity that allows for exquisite specificity, an ability to remember the previous existence

[a] BrightHeart Veterinary Centers, 80 Business Park Drive, Suite 110, Armonk, NY 10504, USA
[b] Memorial Sloan-Kettering Cancer Center, 1275 York Avenue, New York, NY 10065, USA
* Memorial Sloan-Kettering Cancer Center, 1275 York Avenue, New York, NY 10065.
E-mail address: pbergman@brightheartvet.com

Vet Clin Small Anim 40 (2010) 507–518
doi:10.1016/j.cvsm.2010.01.002
0195-5616/10/$ – see front matter © 2010 Elsevier Inc. All rights reserved.

vetsmall.theclinics.com

of the pathogen (ie, memory) and differentiate self from nonself, and the ability to respond more vigorously on repeat exposure to the pathogen. Adaptive immunity consists of T and B lymphocytes. The T cells are further divided into CD8 (cluster of differentiation) & MHC (major histocompatibility complex) Class I cytotoxic helper T cells (CD4 & MHC class II) NK cells, and regulatory T cells. B lymphocytes produce antibodies (humoral system) that may activate complement, enhance phagocytosis of opsonized target cells, and induce antibody-dependent cellular cytotoxicity. B-cell responses to tumors are believed by many investigators to be less important than the development of T cell–mediated immunity, but there is little evidence to fully support this notion.[3] The innate and adaptive arms of immunity are not mutually exclusive; they are linked by (1) the ability of the innate response to stimulate and influence the nature of the adaptive response and (2) the sharing of effector mechanisms between innate and adaptive immune responses.

Immune responses can be further separated by whether they are induced by exposure to a foreign antigen (an active response) or transferred through serum or lymphocytes from an immunized individual (a passive response). Although both approaches have the ability to be extremely specific for an antigen of interest, one important difference is the inability of passive approaches to confer memory. The principal components of the active/adaptive immune system are lymphocytes, antigen-presenting cells, and effector cells. Furthermore, responses can be subdivided by whether they are specific for a certain antigen, or nonspecific, whereby immunity is attempted to be conferred by up-regulating the immune system without a specific target. These definitions are helpful as they allow methodologies to be more completely characterized, such as active-specific, passive-nonspecific, and so forth.

Immune Surveillance

The idea that the immune system may actively prevent the development of neoplasia is termed cancer immunosurveillance. Evidence to support some aspects of this hypothesis[4–7] includes (1) interferon (IFN)-γ protects mice against the growth of tumors, (2) mice lacking IFN-γ receptor are more sensitive to chemically induced sarcomas than normal mice and are more likely to spontaneously develop tumors, (3) mice lacking major components of the adaptive immune response (T and B cells) have a high rate of spontaneous tumors, and (4) mice that lack IFN-γ and B/T cells develop tumors, especially at a young age.

Immune Evasion by Tumors

There are significant barriers to the generation of effective antitumor immunity by the host. Many tumors evade surveillance mechanisms and grow in immunocompetent hosts, which is shown by the large numbers of people and animals succumbing to cancer. There are several ways in which tumors evade the immune response including (1) immunosuppressive cytokine production (eg, tumor growth factor [TGF]-β and interleukin 10 [IL-10])[8,9]; (2) impaired DC function via inactivation (anergy) or poor DC maturation through changes in IL-6/IL-10/vascular endothelial growth factor(VEGF)/granulocyte-macrophage colony-stimulating factor (GM-CSF)[10]; (3) induction of regulatory T cells (Treg), which were initially called suppressor T cells (CD4/CD25/cytotoxic T lymphocyte antigen 4 [CTLA-4]/glucocorticoid-induced tumor necrosis factor receptor family–related gene [GITR]/Foxp3-positive cells, which can suppress tumor-specific CD4/CD8+ T cells)[11]; (4) MHC I loss through structural defects, changes in B2-microglobulin synthesis, defects in transporter-associated antigen processing or actual MHC I gene loss (ie, allelic or locus loss); and (5) MHC I antigen presentation loss through B7-1 attenuation (B7-1 is an important costimulatory molecule for

CD28-mediated T cell receptor and MHC engagement) when the MHC system in #4 remains intact.

NONSPECIFIC TUMOR IMMUNOTHERAPY

In the early 1900s, Dr William Coley, a New York surgeon, noted that some cancer patients who developed incidental bacterial infections survived longer than those without infection.[12] Coley developed a bacterial vaccine (killed cultures of *Serratia marcescens* and *Streptococcus pyogenes* Coley toxins) to treat people with sarcomas that provided complete response rates of approximately 15%. High failure rates and significant side effects led to discontinuation of this approach. His seminal work laid the foundation for nonspecific modulation of the immune response in the treatment of cancer. This article discusses numerous nonspecific tumor immunotherapy approaches, ranging from biologic response modifiers (BRMs) to recombinant cytokines.

BRMs

BRMs are molecules that can modify the biologic response of cells to changes in their external environment, which in the context of cancer immunotherapy could easily span nonspecific and specific immunotherapies. This section discusses nonspecific BRMs (sometimes termed immunopotentiators), which are often related to bacteria or viruses.

One of the earliest BRM discoveries after Coley toxin was the use of bacillus Calmette-Guérin (BCG; Guérin was a veterinarian). BCG is the live attenuated strain of *Mycobacterium bovis*, and intravesical instillation in the urinary bladder causes a significant local inflammatory response that results in antitumor responses.[13] The use of BCG in veterinary patients was first reported by Owen and Bostock[14] in 1974 and has been investigated with numerous types of cancers including urinary bladder carcinoma, osteosarcoma, lymphoma, prostatic carcinoma, transmissible venereal tumor, mammary tumors, sarcoids, squamous cell carcinoma, and others.[15–18] Recently, the use of LDI-100, a product containing BCG and human chorionic gonadotropin (hCG), was compared with vinblastine in dogs with measurable grade II or III mast cell tumors.[19] Response rates were 28.6% and 11.7%, respectively, and the LDI-100 group had significantly less neutropenia. It is particularly exciting for veterinary cancer immunotherapy to potentially be able to use a BRM product that has greater efficacy and less toxicity than a chemotherapy standard of care. However, LDI-100 is not commercially available at present.

Corynebacterium parvum is another BRM which has been investigated for several tumors in veterinary medicine, including melanoma and mammary carcinoma.[20,21] Other bacterially derived BRMs include attenuated *Salmonella typhimurium* (VNP20009), mycobacterial cell wall DNA complexes (MCC; abstracts only at present), and bacterial superantigens.[22,23] Mycobacterial cell walls contain muramyl dipeptide (MDP), which can activate monocytes and tissue macrophages. Muramyl tripeptide phosphatidylethanolamine (MTP-PE) is an analog of MDP. When encapsulated in multilamellar liposomes (L-MTP-PE), monocytes and macrophages uptake MTP leading to activation and subsequent tumoricidal effects through induction of multiple cytokines, including IL-1a, IL-1b, IL-7, IL-8, IL-12, and tumor necrosis factor (TNF).[24] L-MTP-PE has been investigated in numerous tumors in human and veterinary patients, including osteosarcoma, hemangiosarcoma, and mammary carcinoma.[24–28]

Oncolytic viruses have also been used as nonspecific anticancer BRMs in human and veterinary patients.[29] Adenoviruses have been engineered to transcriptionally target canine osteosarcoma cells and have been tested in vitro and in normal dogs with no major signs of virus-associated side effects.[30-32] Similarly, canine distemper virus (CDV), the canine equivalent of human measles virus, has been used in vitro to infect canine lymphocyte cell lines and neoplastic lymphocytes from dogs with B and T cell lymphoma,[33] with high infectivity rates, suggesting that CDV may be investigated in the future for treatment of dogs with lymphoma.

Imiquimod (Aldara) is a novel BRM that is a toll-like receptor 7 (TLR7) agonist.[34] Imiquimod has been reported to be successful in the treatment of Bowen disease (multicentric squamous cell carcinoma in situ) and other skin diseases in humans. Twelve cats with Bowen-like disease were treated topically with imiquimod 5% cream and initial and all subsequent new lesions responded in all cats.[35] An additional cat with pinnal actinic keratoses and squamous cell carcinoma has subsequently been reported to have been successfully treated with topical imiquimod 5% cream.[36] It therefore seems that imiquimod 5% cream is well tolerated in most cats, and further studies are warranted to examine its usefulness in cats and dogs with other skin tumors that are not treatable through standardized means.

Recombinant Cytokines, Growth Factors and Hormones

Several investigations using recombinant cytokines, growth factors, or hormones in various fashions for human and veterinary cancer patients have been reported. Many have investigated the in vitro or in vivo effects of the soluble cytokine (eg, IFNs, IL-2, IL-12, IL-15),[37-48] liposome encapsulation of the cytokine (eg, liposomal IL-2),[38,49-52] or use a virus, cell, liposome-DNA complex, plasmid, or other mechanism to expresses the cytokine (eg, recombinant poxvirus expressing IL-2).[49,53-59]

CANCER VACCINES

The ultimate goal for a cancer vaccine is elicitation of an antitumor immune response that results in clinical regression of a tumor or its metastases. There are numerous types of tumor vaccines in phase I, II, and III trials across a wide range of tumor types. Responses to cancer vaccines may take several months or more to appear because of the slower speed of induction of the adaptive arm of the immune system, as outlined in **Table 1**.

The immune system detects tumors through specific tumor-associated antigens (TAAs) that are recognized by CTLs and antibodies.[60] TAAs may be common to a particular tumor type, be unique to an individual tumor, or may arise from mutated gene products such as ras, p53, or p21. Although unique TAAs may be more immunogenic than the aforementioned shared tumor antigens, they are not practical targets because of their narrow specificity. Most shared tumor antigens are normal cellular antigens that are overexpressed in tumors. The first group to be identified was termed cancer testes antigens because of their expression in normal testes, but they are also

Treatment Type	Mechanism of Action	Specificity	Sensitivity	Response Time	Durability of Response
Chemotherapy	Cytotoxicity	Poor	Variable	Hours to days	Variable
Antitumor vaccine	Immune response	Good	Good	Weeks to months	Variable to long

Table 1
Comparison of chemotherapy and antitumor vaccines

found in melanoma and various other solid tumors such as the MAGE/BAGE gene family. This article highlights those tumor vaccine approaches that seem to hold particular promise in human clinical trials and many that have been tested to date in veterinary medicine.

A variety of approaches have been taken to focus the immune system on the afore-mentioned targets, including (1) whole cell, tumor cell lysate, or subunit vaccines (autologous, or made from a patient's own tumor tissue; allogeneic, or made from individuals within a species bearing the same type of cancer; or whole-cell vaccines from γ-irradiated tumor cell lines with or without immunostimulatory cytokines)[55,61–67]; (2) DNA vaccines that immunize with syngeneic or xenogeneic (different species than recipient) plasmid DNA designed to elicit antigen-specific humoral and cellular immunity[68] (discussed in more detail later in this article); (3) viral vector–based methodologies designed to deliver genes encoding TAAs or immunostimulatory cytokines[69–71]; (4) DC vaccines that are commonly loaded or transfected with TAAs, DNA, or RNA from TAAs, or tumor lysates[72–77]; (5) adoptive cell transfer (the transfer of specific populations of immune effector cells to generate a more powerful and focused antitumor immune response); and (6) antibody approaches such as monoclonal antibodies,[78] anti-idiotype antibodies (an idiotype is an immunoglobulin sequence unique to each B lymphocyte, and therefore antibodies directed against these idiotypes are referred to as anti-idiotype), or conjugated antibodies. The ideal cancer immunotherapy agent would be able to discriminate between cancer and normal cells (ie, specificity), be potent enough to kill small or large numbers of tumor cells (ie, sensitivity), and be able to prevent recurrence of the tumor (ie, durability).

This author has developed a xenogeneic DNA vaccine program for melanoma in collaboration with human investigators from the Memorial Sloan-Kettering Cancer Center.[79,80] Preclinical and clinical studies by our laboratory and others have shown that xenogeneic DNA vaccination with tyrosinase family members (eg, tyrosinase, GP100, GP75) can produce immune responses resulting in tumor rejection or protection and prolongation of survival, whereas syngeneic vaccination with orthologous DNA does not induce immune responses. These studies provided the impetus for development of a xenogeneic DNA vaccine program in canine malignant melanoma (CMM). Cohorts of dogs received increasing doses of xenogeneic plasmid DNA encoding human tyrosinase (huTyr), murine GP75 (muGP75), murine tyrosinase (muTyr), muTyr with or without huGM-CSF (both administered as plasmid DNA) or muTyr off-study intramuscularly biweekly for a total of 4 vaccinations. We and our collaborators have investigated the antibody and T cell responses in dogs vaccinated with huTyr. Antigen-specific (huTyr) IFNγ T cells were found along with two- to fivefold increases in circulating antibodies to huTyr that can cross-react to canine tyrosinase, suggesting the breaking of tolerance.[81,82] The clinical results showing prolongation in survival have been reported previously.[79,80] The results of these trials show that xenogeneic DNA vaccination in CMM (1) is safe, (2) leads to the development of antityrosinase antibodies and T cells, (3) is potentially therapeutic, and (4) is an attractive candidate for further evaluation in an adjuvant, minimal residual disease phase II setting for CMM. The authors and their industrial sponsor, Merial Inc, have completed a multisite US Department of Agriculture safety/efficacy trial of huTyr DNA vaccination in dogs with locoregionally controlled stage II/III oral malignant melanoma. This work has resulted in the receipt of a conditional license for widespread commercial use with the results from the efficacy trial supporting subsequent application for full licensure.[83] Human clinical trials using various xenogeneic melanosomal antigens as DNA (or peptide with adjuvant) vaccination began in 2005, and the preliminary results look favorable.[84–86] To further highlight xenogeneic DNA vaccination as a platform to target other possible antigens for other histologies, the authors have recently completed a phase I trial of murine CD20 for dogs with B cell lymphoma, and will be initiating additional trials such as a phase I trial of rat HER2 and a phase II trial of murine CD20.

Tumor immunology and immunotherapy is one of the most exciting and rapidly expanding fields at present. Significant resources are focused on mechanisms to simultaneously maximally stimulate an antitumor immune response while minimizing the immunosuppressive aspects of the tumor microenvironment.[8] The recent elucidation and blockade of immunosuppressive cytokines (eg, TGF-β, IL-10, and IL-13) or the negative costimulatory molecule CTLA-4,[87,88] along with the functional characterization of T regulatory cells,[89–91] may greatly improve cell-mediated immunity to tumors. As investigators more easily generate specific antitumor immune responses in patients, care is needed to avoid pushing the immune system into pathologic autoimmunity. In addition, immunotherapy is unlikely to become a sole modality in the treatment of cancer, as the traditional modalities of surgery, radiation, or chemotherapy are likely to be used in combination with immunotherapy in the future. Like any form of anticancer treatment, immunotherapy seems to work best in a minimal residual disease setting, suggesting that its most appropriate use will be in an adjuvant setting with local tumor therapies such as surgery or radiation.[92] Similarly, the long-held belief that chemotherapy attenuates immune responses from cancer vaccines is beginning to be disproven through investigations on a variety of levels.[93,94]

SUMMARY

The future looks bright for immunotherapy. The veterinary oncology profession is uniquely able to contribute to the many advances to come in this field. However, what works in a mouse will often not reflect the outcome in human patients with cancer. Therefore, comparative immunotherapy studies using veterinary patients may be better able to bridge murine and human studies. Many cancers in dogs and cats seem to be remarkably stronger models for their counterpart human tumors than presently available murine model systems.[95,96] This is likely due to a variety of reasons including, but not limited to, extreme similarities in the biology of the tumors (eg, chemoresistance, radioresistance, sharing metastatic phenotypes, and site selectivity), spontaneous syngeneic cancer (typically vs an induced or xenogeneic cancer in murine models), and because the dogs and cats that are spontaneously developing these tumors are outbred, immune competent, and live in the same environment as humans. This author looks forward to the time when immunotherapy plays a significant role in the treatment and/or prevention of cancer in human and veterinary patients.

REFERENCES

1. Bergman PJ. Biologic response modification. In: Rosenthal RC, editor. Veterinary oncology secrets. 1st edition. Philadelphia: Hanley & Belfus, Inc; 2001. p. 79–82.
2. Baxevanis CN, Perez SA, Papamichail M. Cancer immunotherapy. Crit Rev Clin Lab Sci 2009;46:167–89.
3. Reilly RT, Emens LA, Jaffee EM. Humoral and cellular immune responses: independent forces or collaborators in the fight against cancer? Curr Opin Investig Drugs 2001;2(1):133–5.
4. Smyth MJ, Godfrey DI, Trapani JA. A fresh look at tumor immunosurveillance and immunotherapy. Nat Immunol 2001;2(4):293–9.

5. Wallace ME, Smyth MJ. The role of natural killer cells in tumor control–effectors and regulators of adaptive immunity. Springer Semin Immunopathol 2005;27(1): 49–64.

6. Itoh H, Horiuchi Y, Nagasaki T, et al. Evaluation of immunological status in tumor-bearing dogs. Vet Immunol Immunopathol 2009;132(2–4):85–90.

7. Schmiedt CW, Grimes JA, Holzman G, et al. Incidence and risk factors for development of malignant neoplasia after feline renal transplantation and cyclosporine-based immunosuppression. Vet Comp Oncol 2009;7:45–53.

8. Catchpole B, Gould SM, Kellett-Gregory LM, et al. Immunosuppressive cytokines in the regional lymph node of a dog suffering from oral malignant melanoma. J Small Anim Pract 2002;43(10):464–7.

9. Zagury D, Gallo RC. Anti-cytokine Ab immune therapy: present status and perspectives. Drug Discov Today 2004;9(2):72–81.

10. Morse MA, Mosca PJ, Clay TM, et al. Dendritic cell maturation in active immunotherapy strategies. Expert Opin Biol Ther 2002;2(1):35–43.

11. Yamaguchi T, Sakaguchi S. Regulatory T cells in immune surveillance and treatment of cancer. Semin Cancer Biol 2006;16(2):115–23.

12. Richardson MA, Ramirez T, Russell NC, et al. Coley toxins immunotherapy: a retrospective review. Altern Ther Health Med 1999;5(3):42–7.

13. Herr HW, Morales A. History of bacillus Calmette-Guerin and bladder cancer: an immunotherapy success story. J Urol 2008;179:53–6.

14. Owen LN, Bostock DE. Proceedings: tumour therapy in dogs using B.C.G. Br J Cancer 1974;29:95.

15. MacEwen EG. An immunologic approach to the treatment of cancer. Vet Clin North Am 1977;7:65–75.

16. Theilen GH, Hills D. Comparative aspects of cancer immunotherapy: immunologic methods used for treatment of spontaneous cancer in animals. J Am Vet Med Assoc 1982;181:1134–41.

17. MacEwen EG. Approaches to cancer therapy using biological response modifiers. Vet Clin North Am Small Anim Pract 1985;15:667–88.

18. Klein WR, Rutten VP, Steerenberg PA, et al. The present status of BCG treatment in the veterinary practice. In Vivo 1991;5:605–8.

19. Henry CJ, Downing S, Rosenthal RC, et al. Evaluation of a novel immunomodulator composed of human chorionic gonadotropin and bacillus Calmette-Guerin for treatment of canine mast cell tumors in clinically affected dogs. Am J Vet Res 2007;68:1246–51.

20. Parodi AL, Misdorp W, Mialot JP, et al. Intratumoral BCG and *Corynebacterium parvum* therapy of canine mammary tumours before radical mastectomy. Cancer Immunol Immunother 1983;15:172–7.

21. MacEwen EG, Patnaik AK, Harvey HJ, et al. Canine oral melanoma: comparison of surgery versus surgery plus *Corynebacterium parvum*. Cancer Invest 1986; 4(5):397–402.

22. Thamm DH, Kurzman ID, King I, et al. Systemic administration of an attenuated, tumor-targeting *Salmonella typhimurium* to dogs with spontaneous neoplasia: phase I evaluation. Clin Cancer Res 2005;11:4827–34.

23. Dow SW, Elmslie RE, Willson AP, et al. In vivo tumor transfection with superantigen plus cytokine genes induces tumor regression and prolongs survival in dogs with malignant melanoma. J Clin Invest 1998;101:2406–14.

24. Kleinerman ES, Jia S-F, Griffin J, et al. Phase II study of liposomal muramyl tripeptide in osteosarcoma: the cytokine cascade and monocyte activation following administration. J Clin Oncol 1992;10:1310–6.

25. MacEwen EG, Kurzman ID, Vail DM, et al. Adjuvant therapy for melanoma in dogs: results of randomized clinical trials using surgery, liposome-encapsulated muramyl tripeptide, and granulocyte macrophage colony-stimulating factor. Clin Cancer Res 1999;5:4249–58.

26. Teske E, Rutteman GR, vd Ingh TS, et al. Liposome-encapsulated muramyl tripeptide phosphatidylethanolamine (L-MTP-PE): a randomized clinical trial in dogs with mammary carcinoma. Anticancer Res 1998;18:1015–9.

27. Kurzman ID, MacEwen EG, Rosenthal RC, et al. Adjuvant therapy for osteosarcoma in dogs: results of randomized clinical trials using combined liposome-encapsulated muramyl tripeptide and cisplatin. Clin Cancer Res 1995;1: 1595–601.

28. Vail DM, MacEwen EG, Kurzman ID, et al. Liposome-encapsulated muramyl tripeptide phosphatidylethanolamine adjuvant immunotherapy for splenic hemangiosarcoma in the dog: a randomized multi-institutional clinical trial. Clin Cancer Res 1995;1:1165–70.

29. Arendt M, Nasir L, Morgan IM. Oncolytic gene therapy for canine cancers: teaching old dog viruses new tricks. Vet Comp Oncol 2009;7:153–61.

30. Smith BF, Curiel DT, Ternovoi VV, et al. Administration of a conditionally replicative oncolytic canine adenovirus in normal dogs. Cancer Biother Radiopharm 2006; 21:601–6.

31. Le LP, Rivera AA, Glasgow JN, et al. Infectivity enhancement for adenoviral transduction of canine osteosarcoma cells. Gene Ther 2006;13:389–99.

32. Hemminki A, Kanerva A, Kremer EJ, et al. A canine conditionally replicating adenovirus for evaluating oncolytic virotherapy in a syngeneic animal model. Mol Ther 2003;7:163–73.

33. Suter SE, Chein MB, von MV, et al. In vitro canine distemper virus infection of canine lymphoid cells: a prelude to oncolytic therapy for lymphoma. Clin Cancer Res 2005;11:1579–87.

34. Meyer T, Stockfleth E. Clinical investigations of toll-like receptor agonists. Expert Opin Investig Drugs 2008;17:1051–65.

35. Gill VL, Bergman PJ, Baer KE, et al. Use of imiquimod 5% cream (Aldara) in cats with multicentric squamous cell carcinoma in situ: 12 cases (2002–2005). Vet Comp Oncol 2008;6:55–64.

36. Peters-Kennedy J, Scott DW, Miller WH Jr. Apparent clinical resolution of pinnal actinic keratoses and squamous cell carcinoma in a cat using topical imiquimod 5% cream. J Feline Med Surg 2008;10(6):593–9.

37. Tateyama S, Priosoeryanto BP, Yamaguchi R, et al. In vitro growth inhibition activities of recombinant feline interferon on all lines derived from canine tumors. Res Vet Sci 1995;59:275–7.

38. Kruth SA. Biological response modifiers: interferons, interleukins, recombinant products, liposomal products. Vet Clin North Am Small Anim Pract 1998;28: 269–95.

39. Whitley EM, Bird AC, Zucker KE, et al. Modulation by canine interferon-gamma of major histocompatibility complex and tumor-associated antigen expression in canine mammary tumor and melanoma cell lines. Anticancer Res 1995;15:923–9.

40. Hampel V, Schwarz B, Kempf C, et al. Adjuvant immunotherapy of feline fibrosarcoma with recombinant feline interferon-omega. J Vet Intern Med 2007;21: 1340–6.

41. Finocchiaro LM, Glikin GC. Cytokine-enhanced vaccine and suicide gene therapy as surgery adjuvant treatments for spontaneous canine melanoma. Gene Ther 2008;15:267–76.

42. Cutrera J, Torrero M, Shiomitsu K, et al. Intratumoral bleomycin and IL-12 electro-chemogenetherapy for treating head and neck tumors in dogs. Methods Mol Biol 2008;423:319–25.

43. Finocchiaro LM, Fiszman GL, Karara AL, et al. Suicide gene and cytokines combined nonviral gene therapy for spontaneous canine melanoma. Cancer Gene Ther 2008;15:165–72.

44. Akhtar N, Padilla ML, Dickerson EB, et al. Interleukin-12 inhibits tumor growth in a novel angiogenesis canine hemangiosarcoma xenograft model. Neoplasia 2004;6:106–16.

45. Dickerson EB, Fosmire S, Padilla ML, et al. Potential to target dysregulated inter-leukin-2 receptor expression in canine lymphoid and hematopoietic malignancies as a model for human cancer. J Immunother 2002;25:36–45.

46. Okano F, Yamada K. Canine interleukin-18 induces apoptosis and enhances Fas ligand mRNA expression in a canine carcinoma cell line. Anticancer Res 2000;20:3411–5.

47. Jahnke A, Hirschberger J, Fischer C, et al. Intra-tumoral gene delivery of feIL-2, feIFN-gamma and feGM-CSF using magnetofection as a neoadjuvant treatment option for feline fibrosarcomas: a phase-I study. J Vet Med A Physiol Pathol Clin Med 2007;54:599–606.

48. Dickerson EB, Akhtar N, Steinberg H, et al. Enhancement of the antiangiogenic activity of interleukin-12 by peptide targeted delivery of the cytokine to alphavbeta3 integrin. Mol Cancer Res 2004;2:663–73.

49. Dow S, Elmslie R, Kurzman I, et al. Phase I study of liposome-DNA complexes encoding the interleukin-2 gene in dogs with osteosarcoma lung metastases. Hum Gene Ther 2005;16:937–46.

50. Skubitz KM, Anderson PM. Inhalational interleukin-2 liposomes for pulmonary metastases: a phase I clinical trial. Anticancer Drugs 2000;11:555–63.

51. Khanna C, Anderson PM, Hasz DE, et al. Interleukin-2 liposome inhalation therapy is safe and effective for dogs with spontaneous pulmonary metastases. Cancer 1997;79:1409–21.

52. Khanna C, Hasz DE, Klausner JS, et al. Aerosol delivery of interleukin 2 liposomes is nontoxic and biologically effective: canine studies. Clin Cancer Res 1996;2:721–34.

53. Jourdier TM, Moste C, Bonnet MC, et al. Local immunotherapy of spontaneous feline fibrosarcomas using recombinant poxviruses expressing interleukin 2 (IL2). Gene Ther 2003;10(26):2126–32.

54. Siddiqui F, Li CY, Zhang X, et al. Characterization of a recombinant adenovirus vector encoding heat-inducible feline interleukin-12 for use in hyperthermia-induced gene-therapy. Int J Hyperthermia 2006;22:117–34.

55. Quintin-Colonna F, Devauchelle P, Fradelizi D, et al. Gene therapy of spontaneous canine melanoma and feline fibrosarcoma by intratumoral administration of histo-incompatible cells expressing human interleukin-2. Gene Ther 1996;3(12):1104–12.

56. Kamstock D, Guth A, Elmslie R, et al. Liposome-DNA complexes infused intrave-nously inhibit tumor angiogenesis and elicit antitumor activity in dogs with soft tissue sarcoma. Cancer Gene Ther 2006;13:306–17.

57. Junco JA, Basalto R, Fuentes F, et al. Gonadotrophin releasing hormone-based vaccine, an effective candidate for prostate cancer and other hormone-sensitive neoplasms. Adv Exp Med Biol 2008;617:581–7.

58. Chou PC, Chuang TF, Jan TR, et al. Effects of immunotherapy of IL-6 and IL-15 plasmids on transmissible venereal tumor in beagles. Vet Immunol Immunopathol 2009;130(1–2):25–34.

59. Chuang TF, Lee SC, Liao KW, et al. Electroporation-mediated IL-12 gene therapy in a transplantable canine cancer model. Int J Cancer 2009;125(3):698–707.

60. Bergman PJ. Anticancer vaccines. Vet Clin North Am Small Anim Pract 2007;37: 1111–9.

61. Hogge GS, Burkholder JK, Culp J, et al. Preclinical development of human granulocyte-macrophage colony-stimulating factor-transfected melanoma cell vaccine using established canine cell lines and normal dogs. Cancer Gene Ther 1999;6(1):26–36.

62. Alexander AN, Huelsmeyer MK, Mitzey A, et al. Development of an allogeneic whole-cell tumor vaccine expressing xenogeneic gp100 and its implementation in a phase II clinical trial in canine patients with malignant melanoma. Cancer Immunol Immunother 2006;55(4):433–42.

63. U'Ren LW, Biller BJ, Elmslie RE, et al. Evaluation of a novel tumor vaccine in dogs with hemangiosarcoma. J Vet Intern Med 2007;21:113–20.

64. Bird RC, Deinnocentes P, Lenz S, et al. An allogeneic hybrid-cell fusion vaccine against canine mammary cancer. Vet Immunol Immunopathol 2008; 123:289–304.

65. Turek MM, Thamm DH, Mitzey A, et al. Human granulocyte & macrophage colony-stimulating factor DNA cationic-lipid complexed autologous tumour cell vaccination in the treatment of canine B-cell multicentric lymphoma. Vet Comp Oncol 2007;5:219–31.

66. Kuntsi-Vaattovaara H, Verstraete FJM, Newsome JT, et al. Resolution of persistent oral papillomatosis in a dog after treatment with a recombinant canine oral papillomavirus vaccine. Vet Comp Oncol 2003;1:57–63.

67. Milner RJ, Salute M, Crawford C, et al. The immune response to disialoganglioside GD3 vaccination in normal dogs: a melanoma surface antigen vaccine. Vet Immunol Immunopathol 2006;114:273–84.

68. Kamstock D, Elmslie R, Thamm D, et al. Evaluation of a xenogeneic VEGF vaccine in dogs with soft tissue sarcoma. Cancer Immunol Immunother 2007; 56:1299–309.

69. von EH, Sadeghi A, Carlsson B, et al. Efficient adenovector CD40 ligand immunotherapy of canine malignant melanoma. J Immunother 2008;31:377–84.

70. Johnston KB, Monteiro JM, Schultz LD, et al. Protection of beagle dogs from mucosal challenge with canine oral papillomavirus by immunization with recombinant adenoviruses expressing codon-optimized early genes. Virology 2005;336:208–18.

71. Thacker EE, Nakayama M, Smith BF, et al. A genetically engineered adenovirus vector targeted to CD40 mediates transduction of canine dendritic cells and promotes antigen-specific immune responses in vivo. Vaccine 2009;27(50): 7116–24.

72. Gyorffy S, Rodriguez-Lecompte JC, Woods JP, et al. Bone marrow-derived dendritic cell vaccination of dogs with naturally occurring melanoma by using human gp100 antigen. J Vet Intern Med 2005;19(1):56–63.

73. Tamura K, Arai H, Ueno E, et al. Comparison of dendritic cell-mediated immune responses among canine malignant cells. J Vet Med Sci 2007;69: 925–30.

74. Tamura K, Yamada M, Isotani M, et al. Induction of dendritic cell-mediated immune responses against canine malignant melanoma cells. Vet J 2008;175: 126–9.

75. Rodriguez-Lecompte JC, Kruth S, Gyorffy S, et al. Cell-based cancer gene therapy: breaking tolerance or inducing autoimmunity? Anim Health Res Rev 2004;5:227–34.

76. Kyte JA, Mu L, Aamdal S, et al. Phase I/II trial of melanoma therapy with dendritic cells transfected with autologous tumor-mRNA. Cancer Gene Ther 2006;13:905–18.

77. Mason NJ, Coughlin CM, Overley B, et al. RNA-loaded CD40-activated B cells stimulate antigen-specific T-cell responses in dogs with spontaneous lymphoma. Gene Ther 2008;15:955–65.

78. Jeglum KA. Chemoimmunotherapy of canine lymphoma with adjuvant canine monoclonal antibody 231. Vet Clin North Am Small Anim Pract 1996;26(1):73–85.

79. Bergman PJ, Camps-Palau MA, McKnight JA, et al. Development of a xenogeneic DNA vaccine program for canine malignant melanoma at the Animal Medical Center. Vaccine 2006;24(21):4582–5.

80. Bergman PJ, McKnight J, Novosad A, et al. Long-term survival of dogs with advanced malignant melanoma after DNA vaccination with xenogeneic human tyrosinase: a phase I trial. Clin Cancer Res 2003;9(4):1284–90.

81. Liao JC, Gregor P, Wolchok JD, et al. Vaccination with human tyrosinase DNA induces antibody responses in dogs with advanced melanoma. Cancer Immun 2006;6:8.

82. Goubier A, Fuhrmann L, Forest L, et al. Superiority of needle-free transdermal plasmid delivery for the induction of antigen-specific IFNgamma T cell responses in the dog. Vaccine 2008;26:2186–90.

83. Bergman PJ, Wolchok JD. Of mice and men (and dogs): development of a xenogeneic DNA vaccine for canine oral malignant melanoma. Cancer Ther 2008;6:817–26.

84. Wolchok JD, Yuan J, Houghton AN, et al. Safety and immunogenicity of tyrosinase DNA vaccines in patients with melanoma. Mol Ther 2007;15:2044–50.

85. Perales MA, Yuan J, Powel S, et al. Phase I/II study of GM-CSF DNA as an adjuvant for a multipeptide cancer vaccine in patients with advanced melanoma. Mol Ther 2008;16:2022–9.

86. Yuan J, Ku GY, Gallardo HF, et al. Safety and immunogenicity of a human and mouse gp100 DNA vaccine in a phase I trial of patients with melanoma. Cancer Immun 2009;9:5.

87. Peggs KS, Quezada SA, Korman AJ, et al. Principles and use of anti-CTLA4 antibody in human cancer immunotherapy. Curr Opin Immunol 2006;18(2):206–13.

88. Graves SS, Stone D, Loretz C, et al. Establishment of long-term tolerance to SRBC in dogs by recombinant canine CTLA4-Ig. Transplantation 2009;88:317–22.

89. Biller BJ, Elmslie RE, Burnett RC, et al. Use of FoxP3 expression to identify regulatory T cells in healthy dogs and dogs with cancer. Vet Immunol Immunopathol 2007;116:69–78.

90. Horiuchi Y, Tominaga M, Ichikawa M, et al. Increase of regulatory T cells in the peripheral blood of dogs with metastatic tumors. Microbiol Immunol 2009;53:468–74.

91. O'Neill K, Guth A, Biller B, et al. Changes in regulatory T cells in dogs with cancer and associations with tumor type. J Vet Intern Med 2009;23:875–81.

92. Thamm DH. Interactions between radiation therapy and immunotherapy: the best of two worlds? Vet Comp Oncol 2006;4:189–97.

93. Walter CU, Biller BJ, Lana SE, et al. Effects of chemotherapy on immune responses in dogs with cancer. J Vet Intern Med 2006;20(2):342–7.

94. Emens LA, Jaffee EM. Leveraging the activity of tumor vaccines with cytotoxic chemotherapy. Cancer Res 2005;65(18):8059–64.
95. Khanna C, London C, Vail D, et al. Guiding the optimal translation of new cancer treatments from canine to human cancer patients. Clin Cancer Res 2009;15: 5671–7.
96. Paoloni M, Khanna C. Translation of new cancer treatments from pet dogs to humans. Nat Rev Cancer 2008;8:147–56.

Index

Note: Page numbers of article titles are in **boldface** type.

A

Acrodermatitis, lethal, in bull terriers, 430
Acute immunologic transfusion reactions, 489–490
Acute lung injury, transfusion-related, in small animal practice, 490
Acute nonimmunologic transfusion reactions, in small animal practice, 490–491
Adaptive immunity, 372
Age, immunosuppression in dogs and cats related to, 464–465
Air embolism, transfusion-related, in small animal practice, 491
Allergic reactions, transfusion-related, in small animal practice, 489
Amino acids, immunosuppression in dogs and cats related to, 460
Anaplasma phagocytophilium infection, immunodeficiencies due to, 417–418
Anemia, hemolytic, immmune-mediated, in small animals, 443–444
Anesthesia/anesthetics, immunosuppression in dogs and cats related to, 461–462
Antibody(ies), structure of, in transfusion medicine, in small animal practice, 485–486
Antigen encounter, 373–374
Antinuclear antibody test
    in autoimmune disease detection in small animals, 450–451
    in immunologic disease evaluation in small animals, 470
Aplasia, thymic, hypotrichosis with, in Birman kittens, 430
Arthritis, rheumatoid, in small animals, 449–450
Autoantibody(ies), organ-specific, in autoimmune diseases in small animals,
    detection of, 451–452
Autoimmune diseases, in small animals, **439–457**
    described, 439–440
    detection of, laboratory methods in, 450–452
    diabetes mellitus, 446
    organ system–specific diseases, 443
    SLE, 440–443
    systemic diseases, 440–450
        endocrine, 445–446
        hematologic, 443–445
        musculoskeletal, 448–450
        ocular, 450
        skin, 446–448
    treatment of, approaches to, 452–453
Autoimmune thyroiditis, in small animals, 445–446
Azathioprine, immunosuppression in dogs and cats related to, 462

B

Bacterial infections, immunodeficiencies due to, 416–418
  Anaplasma phagocytophilium infection, 417–418
  described, 416

Vet Clin Small Anim 40 (2010) 519–527
doi:10.1016/S0195-5616(10)00047-1
0195-5616/10/$ – see front matter © 2010 Elsevier Inc. All rights reserved.

vetsmall.theclinics.com

Moving?

Make sure your subscription moves with you!

To notify us of your new address, find your **Clinics Account Number** (located on your mailing label above your name), and contact customer service at:

Email: journalscustomerservice-usa@elsevier.com

800-654-2452 (subscribers in the U.S. & Canada)
314-447-8871 (subscribers outside of the U.S. & Canada)

Fax number: 314-447-8029

Elsevier Health Sciences Division
Subscription Customer Service
3251 Riverport Lane
Maryland Heights, MO 63043

*To ensure uninterrupted delivery of your subscription, please notify us at least 4 weeks in advance of move.

Printed and bound by CPI Group (UK) Ltd, Croydon, CR0 4YY

03/10/2024

01040446-0016